Contents

- Developments in fetal heart rate monitoring
- A brief historical overview of how the fetal heart rate has been monitored
- An introductory discussion concerning the efficacy of electronic fetal heart monitoring
- Present methods of fetal heart rate monitoring
- Correct care and use of equipment
- Checklist for electronic fetal heart rate monitoring

- Physiology related to the fetal heart rate
- Factors which influence fetal oxygenation
- Fetal hypoxia
- Effects of uterine contractions on fetal oxygenation

- Indications for using electronic fetal monitoring antenatally and during labour
- Characteristics of a normal fetal heart rate trace: variability; beat to beat variation; sleep periods; accelerations
- Principles of obtaining an accurate trace and troubleshooting
- Use of telemetry

- Causes of various suspicious and pathological traces
- Midwife's role and responsibilities
- Classification summarizing the range of abnormal fetal heart traces and the action recommended

List of Illustrations

Explanatory Note

The authors discussed at length the positioning of Chapter 6 *Antenatal Electronic Monitoring*. Logic indicated that chronologically this chapter should precede the discussion on labour (chapters 3 and 4). However, the authors felt that antenatal electronic fetal heart monitoring belongs with the abnormal and should follow the discussion on normal, suspicious and abnormal traces in labour. Therefore, the reader should be able to see the progression from normal to increasingly abnormal traces.

Acknowledgements

Many people have helped us with this venture – some wittingly and others unwittingly – we would like to thank them for their involvement.

We are grateful to the midwifery managers (Margaret Stockwell and Lynn Woods) and all the consultants at both the Maternity Units in Leicester for their permission to find and use traces. We would also like to thank the midwives at both units who identified and notified us of interesting traces. Many thanks are also given to the staff of the Maternity Medical Records Departments who have always found time to help us in the search for notes. We recommend their detective work.

We would like to acknowledge the help and support of our husbands for their patience while we have spent evenings and weekends poring over traces and manuscript, without them we would not have found either the time or the energy to write this book. We would also like to acknowledge our children who have had somewhat preoccupied mothers during the process of writing this book. Thanks also go to Mona and Gerald.

To Jill Bentley, Librarian, for all her efforts in obtaining literature and aiding literature searches.

Great thanks are due to our two expert proof readers, Mr Charles Stewart from Leicester (a great supporter of midwives autonomy) and Dr Pauline Hurley from Oxford, both of whose help and advice was greatly appreciated.

Preface

At present the book market has a wide range of texts on fetal heart rate monitoring. It is reasonable, therefore, to ask what has *this* book to offer.

This book has been written with the clinical midwife very much in mind. It is intended to provide material which is helpful when used in the clinical situation and information which can be found easily. The text has been written in a format which is easy to read whilst being up to date and using appropriate references.

Theoretical teaching on fetal heart rate monitoring is now an integral part of the midwifery education curriculum. This book will be a useful guide for putting this knowledge into practice and will be useful to a wide range of qualified midwives as well as students. Some sections may be used as revision, others provide consolidation of knowledge.

Thus the aims of this book are to:

- Provide the midwife/student midwife with information which can easily be utilized in the clinical situation.

- Offer information to a diverse audience ranging from midwives who are being initially introduced to the subject to those who are knowlegeable about fetal heart rate monitoring in clinical practice.

- Consider the related physiology which influences the fetal heart rate.

- Examine a wide range of normal and abnormal fetal heart traces and the midwife's responsibilities in each instance.

- Discuss and debate the use of fetal heart rate monitoring in midwifery and obstetrics; the potential and actual effects of its use will be considered along with future developments.

The text is supported by a wide range of fetal heart traces and a reference section and most chapters are summarized with key facts. At the end of the book there is a recommended reading list to aid further study of fetal monitoring. A glossary is included for easy reference of terms.

CHAPTER ONE

Fetal Heart Rate Monitoring - An Introduction

In the 1990s the search continues to discover equipment which will provide optimum quality information about fetal well-being. This has been the aim since the last century when the fetal heart was first heard through the woman's abdomen. However, regardless of how technology improves, perfect outcomes can never be guaranteed.

Therefore, this chapter considers:

- a brief historical perspective of the developments in monitoring of the fetal heart.

- the present methods of monitoring the fetal heart rate including the correct use and care of the equipment.

- an introduction to the debate concerning the efficacy and reliability of electronic fetal heart rate monitoring.

- an outline of current developments in alternative methods of assessing fetal well being.

An historical perspective

It is reported that no written records existed about fetal life in utero until the 17th century in Western literature (Gibb and Arulkumaran,1992).

	Chronology of events
1818	Francois-Isaac Mayor of Geneva, a surgeon, reported that he could hear the fetal heart by placing his ear against the woman's abdomen. He identified it as being different from the maternal pulse.
1827	John Creery Ferguson was the first person in the British Isles to describe fetal heart sounds. Gibb and Arulkumaran (1992) describe how there was much debate over the most appropriate technique of listening to the fetal heart. Some doctors insisted on using a stethoscope for reasons of decency, some even listened through women's clothing!

1849	Kilian proposed the indications for performing a forceps delivery following fetal stethoscope findings. He suggested that forceps needed to be applied without delay if the fetal heart decreases to less than 100 beats per minute or if it rises to greater than 180 beats per minute or if the beats lost their 'purity of tone'.
1876	Pinard produced his own version of a fetal stethoscope. (Several versions from others had preceded Pinard's own)
1893	Winkel empirically set the limits of the normal fetal heart rate range at 120–160 beats per minute.

It became increasingly recognized that by auscultating the fetal heart intermittently the assessment of its rate was based on a short period of time. This potentially resulted in considerable listener variability. It was felt that more continuous monitoring was desirable. (This remains questionable for low risk clients.)

1958	Hon pioneered electronic fetal monitoring in the USA. Caldeyro-Barcia in Uruguay and Hammacher in Germany reported their observations on various heart rate patterns associated with fetal distress.
1966	Saling in Berlin reported the use of fetal blood sampling to study fetal pH. Fetal scalp blood pH assessment was developed alongside electronic monitoring and not afterwards as current practice seems to indicate.
1968	First fetal monitor by Hammacher and Hewlett Packard. Sonicaid produced their own in the UK shortly afterwards.

Initially phonocardiography was used to listen to and record the sounds coming from the maternal abdomen. This produced poor quality traces due to interference from other sounds. However, the introduction of Doppler ultrasound transducers in 1964 improved the quality of traces. Indeed the improved technology of cardiotocographs enables them to produce excellent quality external traces. (see Fig. 1.1)

The early difficulties with external monitoring of twins has also been resolved with new equipment which uses two different frequencies so that ultrasound beams do not interfere with each other. (see Fig. 1.2.)

Electronic Monitoring of the Fetal Heart

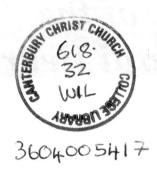

Published by Books for Midwives Press, 174a Ashley Road, Hale, Cheshire, WA15 9SF, England

© 1996, Jacqui Williams and Joanne Blanchard
First edition

ISBN 1-898507-11-2

British Library Cataloguing in Publication Data
A catalogue record for this book is available from the British Library

Printed in Great Britain

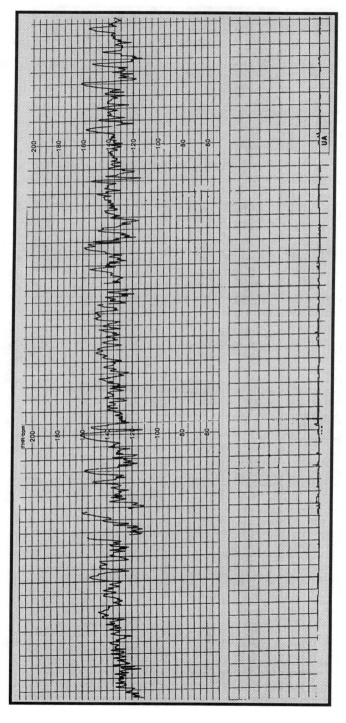

Fig. 1.1: Normal trace using external transducer

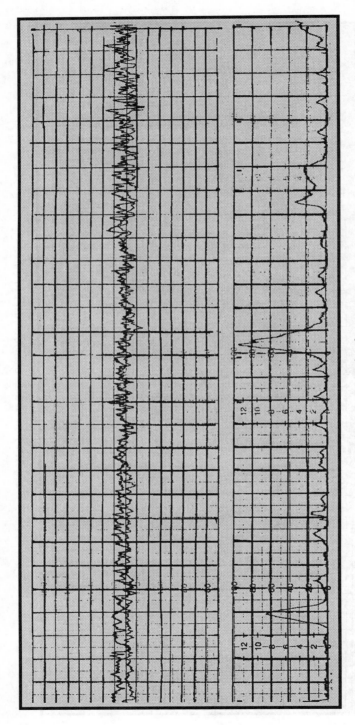

Fig. 1.2: Example of a twin trace

Methods of monitoring the fetal heart rate

The methods of monitoring the fetal heart rate are:

- Intermittent auscultation
  - Pinard's stethoscope
  - doppler ultrasound device

- Continuous fetal heart monitoring
  - electronic fetal monitoring

For all methods of monitoring the fetal heart the midwife must ensure that:

- the woman is prepared for what is going to happen and has given her consent
- the woman feels comfortable and has emptied her bladder recently
- privacy is preserved especially in a hospital environment – only the abdomen needs to be exposed
- an abdominal examination is performed paying particular attention to the position where it would be expected that the fetal heart would be heard.

Intermittent auscultation

The fetal heart can be first heard using a Pinard's stethoscope at 18–24 weeks gestation but as early as 12 weeks gestation with a doppler ultrasound device. Using either method and listening for one minute it is possible to find out whether the fetal heart rate is within normal range (110–150 beats per minute) and that it is regular in nature.

Some practical considerations:

- A metal Pinard's stethoscope, if being used, needs to be warmed to aid the woman's comfort

- The doppler ultrasound needs to be charged and have contact gel smeared on the underside of the transducer. After switching on, the transducer is pressed over the area where the fetal heart is expected to be heard and the volume adjusted to a comfortable level. On completion all traces of the contact gel are wiped off the woman's abdomen.

Intermittent auscultation of the fetal heart is widely available and easy to use. It is non-invasive and inexpensive and is very appropriate for normal antenatal examinations and labours. Intermittent auscultation has been shown to be effective if performed in a consistent manner by one carer at regular intervals appropriate to the stage of labour. It is usually performed for one minute after a contraction. In established labour this is generally done at 15 minute intervals. During the second stage of labour the fetal heart needs to be listened to at five minute intervals. In order to assess the response of the fetal heart rate pattern it needs to be listened to before, during and after a contraction.

Unfortunately busy units may view this as a very labour-intensive method and may not wish to commit staff to provide it (Tucker, 1992). Nevertheless, as the recording of the fetal heart is intermittent and cannot assess variability, continuous fetal heart monitoring may be more appropriate in high risk situations.

There are some instances, however, when using a Pinard's stethoscope would not be appropriate and these are listed below.

• Prior to 24 weeks gestation.

• If there is difficulty hearing the fetal heart because of obesity in the woman.

• If there is any uncertainty about whether the fetal heart can be heard or any concern over its rate or pattern.

• If the woman would like to hear the fetal heart.

One of the advantages of using an intermittent ultrasound device is the pleasure that women and their partners experience in being able to hear the fetal heartbeat. It is also possible to listen to the fetal heart whilst the woman adopts whichever position she chooses, unlike the Pinard's stethoscope which requires the woman to adopt a supine position, possibly predisposing to supine hypotension syndrome.

The efficacy and reliability of electronic fetal heart rate monitoring

Electronic fetal heart rate monitoring (EFM) is frequently used antenatally and in labour to establish fetal well-being. Unfortunately because there is often an insufficient ratio of midwives to clients the use of EFM has served to increase staff productivity where midwives can care for more than one woman at a time. This is a worrying issue. Tucker (1992) suggests that it is unlikely that further advances in high technology equipment will be able to further decrease infant mortality in the future. He proposes that *all* mothers and infants need access to early maternity and paediatric care. Indeed studies to date still demonstrate that intermittent auscultation of low-risk women is as effective as EFM at predicting perinatal outcome (Paine et al, 1992). In any event even if outcomes may be improved by using high technology equipment perfect outcomes can *never* be guaranteed.

Being able to monitor continuously the fetal heart rate has provided us with the opportunity to observe warning signs of fetal compromise. However, controversy still exists about this because randomized trials examining continuous fetal heart rate monitoring cannot demonstrate an improvement in the perinatal mortality rate. In fact, its use accompanies a rise in operative deliveries, although this is reduced where abnormal findings are investigated using fetal blood sampling (Spencer,1992). The studies which have explored the use of EFM have observed that its use is accompanied by a reduction in neonatal seizures (Thacker,1991). Nonetheless, Grant et al (1989) argue that whilst neonatal seizures may be reduced when electronic fetal monitoring is used, cerebral palsy rates have changed little over the last 30 years during which time continuous monitoring has been introduced. It is likely that preventable intrapartum asphyxia is much less common than previously thought. It is probable that long-term cerebral palsy is secondary to some abnormality in the developing fetus.

To date therefore, there is no evidence to indicate that continuous fetal heart rate monitoring is superior to intermittent auscultation particularly in normal midwifery care. It had been hoped that the diagnosing of intrapartum asphyxia would have improved neonatal outcome, however, this has not been the case. This is not simply a problem of electronic fetal heart rate monitoring but of the many ways used to assess neonatal outcome. For example, should Apgar scores be considered or admissions to the neonatal unit or estimation of cord gases. All have their merits and related problems. However, where continuous fetal monitoring does play a part in care of complicated labours, it needs to be supported by further tests and investigations for example, fetal blood sampling, acoustic stimulation. This is vital so that a total picture is considered rather than taking action on insufficient information. The midwife needs to have the knowledge to use appropriately and interpret the equipment and the information it is providing. This is considered in more detail in later chapters but first a look at the choice of equipment that may be used for monitoring the fetal heart would be appropriate.

Current developments

The problems associated with EFM have promoted the search for alternative methods of assessing fetal well-being. These include:

- Electrocardiographic (ECG) waveform analysis
- Systolic time intervals
- Pulse oximetry
- Infrared spectroscopy

Electrocardiographic (ECG) waveform analysis

Changes in the fetal ECG wave patterns have been considered as a potential means of identifying fetal hypoxia since about 1971 (Symonds, 1971). Fetal hypoxia had already been identified to be an indicator of myocardial hypoxaemia in adults (Kahn and Simonson, 1957). The theory behind ECG waveform analysis is based on the fact that the QRS complex represents passive activity of the heart which does not utilize energy unlike the ST waveform. In hypoxic conditions there is an increase in the T:QRS ratio. Several researchers have tried to develop an accurate means of identifying the ST waveform and any changes occurring in relation to the T:QRS ratio and hypoxia (Murphy, Russell and Johnson, 1992; Murray, 1986; Rosen et al, 1986). As yet the technology is still being developed and no conclusions have been reached.

Systolic time intervals

This is another method of assessing fetal wellbeing. Research has included the measurement of the component time intervals of the fetal cardiac cycle, most commonly the pre-ejection period (Organ et al, 1974). The relationship between changes in systolic time intervals and hypoxia have been considered (Hon et al, 1974). As yet, these methods have not been adequately evaluated and technical improvements in the equipment are needed.

Pulse oximetry

Pulse oximeters can record both the heart rate and arterial oxygen saturation and have been used to monitor fetal wellbeing (McNamara et al, 1992; Johnson et al, 1991). However their use is limited at present because of the difficulty of obtaining accurate results due to caput and fetal hair. There is also a wide normal fetal range and further technical development and evaluation is needed. Similar problems have been found with continuous pH measurements.

Infrared spectroscopy

Near infrared spectroscopy (NIRS) utilizes the optical absorption characteristics of oxyhaemoglobin, which are different from those of haemoglobin which is not oxygenated. An optrode is attached to the fetal skull when the cervix is 3cms dilated and the membranes therefore have to be ruptured. The technique uses near infrared light which readily passes through tissues, including the fetal skull and brain. Changes in cerebral blood flow and oxygenation can be identified as they occur. Real-time information relating to what is happening inside the fetal brain can be obtained. The relationship between neonatal outcome and NIRS patterns has not yet been identified. The NIRS pattern of fetuses who have experienced hypoxic episodes before labour commences have also yet to be identified (O'Brien, Doyle and Rolfe, 1993).

Electronic fetal monitoring (EFM)

There are instances when continuous fetal monitoring is more appropriate than intermittently listening to the fetal heart.

Aims of EFM

*   To provide a continuous graphical record of the fetal heart rate and pattern.

*   To be able to observe the response of the fetal heart rate pattern to uterine activity and/or fetal movements.

*   To be an integrated part of care particularly where there is an increased risk of fetal compromise.

It is only in the last 25 years that a useful association has been made between uterine contractions and the fetal heart (although midwives have probably known this instinctively for some time!).

Indications for its use can be divided into antenatal and labour.

Antenatal uses of continuous fetal monitoring

- To monitor fetal well-being in high-risk pregnancies. Examples include raised blood pressure, multiple pregnancy, poor obstetric history i.e. previous stillbirth, intrauterine death, antepartum haemorrhage, multiple pregnancy, suspected preterm labour. A 20–60 minute continuous fetal heart trace may be carried out on a regular basis in high-risk pregnancies to complement antenatal care.

- For suspected antenatal problems, such as reduced fetal movements and weight loss, continuous fetal monitoring may be carried out to accompany a range of other investigative tests.

Use of continuous fetal monitoring during labour

- As requested by the mother.

- For high-risk labours, for example preterm, multiple pregnancies, meconium-stained liquor, intrauterine growth retardation, preeclampsia.

- When labour is being induced using oxytocic preparations.

- When an epidural is in progress.

- Alterations in the fetal heart rate or pattern.

When the fetal heart is monitored continuously it is done by using electronic equipment called cardiotocography (CTG). CTG is the graphical representation of the fetal heart rate and the uterine contractions. EFM can either be performed externally or internally. However, in spite of improved technology a debate still continues over the use of electronic fetal heart monitoring

KEY POINTS

- No written records in Western literature existed about fetal life in utero until the 17th century.

- Following the development of a fetal stethoscope it became increasingly recognized that the rate recorded by auscultating the fetal heart intermittently is based on a short period of time. Intermittent auscultation is subject to considerable listener variability.

- Improved technology has greatly improved the quality of traces.

- The debate continues over the efficiency and reliability of EFM as intermittent auscultation is effective for normal care for detecting fetal heart rate changes if performed in a consistent manner by one carer.

- Current developments continue to search for methods of assessing fetal wellbeing on account of the problems associated with EFM.

CHAPTER TWO

An Outline of the Physiology of the Fetal Heart Rate and Hypoxia

<u>Fetal heart rate patterns change in response to an inadequate supply of oxygen</u> (Hon, 1968; Itskovitz et al, 1982). It is this change in fetal heart rate patterns on which the rationale for electronic fetal heart rate monitoring is based. The purpose, therefore, is to detect at an early stage insufficient oxygenation before permanent damage is done.

Control of the fetal heart rate is very complex and involves many intricate mechanisms. This chapter only provides an introduction to the control of the fetal heart rate and covers the principles rather than all the specific details. Uterine contractions are also considered because of their potential hypoxic effects. This chapter therefore considers:

- Factors which influence fetal oxygenation.
- The effects of the sympathetic nervous system on fetal heart rate.
- The effects of the parasympathetic nervous system on fetal heart rate.
- The role of the baroreceptors and chemoreceptors in the control of the fetal heart rate.
- The effect of insufficient oxygen on cardiac function.
- The ability of the fetus to compensate for insufficient oxygen.
- The effect of uterine contractions on fetal oxygenation.

Fetal hypoxia can occur at any gestational age. It can be acute as in placental abruption or chronic as in placental insufficiency.

Fetal oxygenation is dependent on:
1) maternal oxygenation
2) maternal blood flow
3) placental function
4) fetal circulation

Fetal hypoxia can therefore be due to inadequate oxygenation of the mother or inadequate blood flow (maternal or fetal in origin) or both as in maternal smoking (Williams et al 1993; Christianson, 1979).

Fetal circulation is reliant on fetal cardiac output. Cardiac activity is reliant on oxygenation.

Cardiac output = Heart Rate x Stroke Volume

The fetal cardiac output, unlike that of adults, is controlled to a great extent by heart rate (Harvey, 1989). Therefore when the fetal heart rate drops cardiac output falls (Rudolph and Heyman, 1976) and with insufficient cardiac output oxygen is not transported to the vital organs.

The heartbeat arises from the sinoatrial node which has an intrinsic rate (Walker, 1984). The rate can be adjusted by the autonomic nervous system both the sympathetic and parasympathetic. When the sympathetic nervous system is stimulated it *increases* the heart rate. When the parasympathetic nervous system is stimulated it acts quickly via the vagal nerve and *decreases* the fetal heart rate (Warner and Cox, 1962). The sympathetic nervous system develops earlier in fetal life than the parasympathetic. Therefore the fetal heart rate is higher in early pregnancy – about 180 bpm at 15 weeks and 150 at 30 weeks (Walker, 1984).

There is continuous interplay between the two systems and this results in the baseline variation or variability of the fetal heart rate. Good baseline variability demonstrates a functional and healthy autonomic nervous system (Kubli and Hon, 1969). When, therefore, the fetal heat rate decelerates, the cardiac output diminishes, oxygenation is inhibited and baseline variability decreases (Smith et al, 1988; Martin, 1982).

The fetal heart rate is modulated by a number of complex mechanisms. The autonomic nervous system concerned with cardiac function is controlled by the cardioregulatory centre in the mid-brain, the medulla oblongata. This centre is in turn influenced by the higher centres of the brain. Other major influences on the heart rate include the chemoreceptors and the baroreceptors (Walker, 1984).

The chemoreceptors are found in the aorta and in the mid-brain. The chemoreceptors are sensitive to oxygen and carbon dioxide tension. A drop in oxygen tension results in the chemoreceptors stimulating sympathetic activity via the cardioregulatory centre and the release of adrenaline. Thus the heart rate would increase. If the drop in oxygen is severe enough blood will be directed to the vital organs (the heart and the brain) and away from the gut, liver and kidneys.

The baroreceptors are found in the large arteries and the aorta. They are stretch receptors and sensitive to arterial blood pressure. When there is a rise in blood pressure (e.g. cord compression) the baroreceptors stimulate parasympathetic activity via the cardioregulatory centre and vagal nerve (Steer, 1990).

If oxygen levels continue to drop, cardiac output will decrease due to a lack of cardiac oxygenation. However, the blood pressure rises in an attempt to compensate for a decreased cardiac output. The baroreceptors recognize the change in blood pressure and thus the parasympathetic nervous system stimulates the vagus nerve causing a decrease in heart rate (Itskovitz, Goetzman and Rudolph, 1982).

It should not be forgotten that both the normal well grown fetus and the new baby (which have not been chronically deprived of oxygen) are fairly resilient to hypoxia. The healthy placenta is more than capable of meeting normal fetal oxygen demands. The transport of oxygen to the fetus appears, in fact, to be more than sufficient. The fetus has a comparatively low arterial pO2 (Williams et al, 1993). The fetus also has high levels of haemoglobin, which has a greater oxygen affinity. In addition the design of the fetal circulation results in a relatively high cardiac output. The fetal environment enables the fetus to develop in a relatively hypoxic environment, where normally oxygen availability exceeds oxygen requirements (Richardson, 1989).

The initial response to a fall in oxygen saturation that is mild or slow to fall is to compensate by triggering sympathetic activity. The fetal heart rate therefore increases in an attempt to increase cardiac output, giving rise to baseline tachycardia. This initial increase in fetal heart rate in response to hypoxia is not necessarily related to fetal acidosis unless there are other signs of fetal compromise such as decelerations and/or a decrease in variability (Steer, 1990; Gibb and Arulkumaran, 1992). Oxygen is necessary to utilize glucose for energy. Oxygen and energy are therefore necessary for the whole nervous system to function adequately, and indeed for all bodily functions. When there is a prolonged lack of oxygen, liver glycogen is mobilized in an attempt to provide an alternative energy source. Glycogen is anaerobically metabolized and therefore causes acidosis with the build-up of lactic acid (Carter, 1993). However, acidosis inhibits cardiac muscle function. The length of time a fetus can withstand hypoxia is dependent on its glycogen reserves. Therefore growth-retarded babies are more susceptible to hypoxia because they have little by way of glycogen reserve (Steer, 1989).

The fetal heart rate and variability may also be affected by numerous other factors. These factors include such things as fetal activity and sleep states (Spencer and Johnson, 1986) and maternal drugs, e.g. benzodiazepines, opiates, beta-blockers and atropine (Whittle, 1988) and maternal conditions, e.g. thyrotoxicosis (Robinson et al, 1979), myxodema (Reginals and Mackinnon, 1984) and a variety of congenital abnormalities of the fetal heart (Maxwell et al, 1988).

One of the aims of monitoring the fetal heart in labour is to prevent fetal hypoxia and thus an asphyxiated baby at delivery. Unfortunately there is no universal definition of birth asphyxia. The causes of cerebral palsy and the role hypoxia plays have not been established. Neither has a test yet been developed which will identify the exact stage at which the hypoxia can permanently affect a fetus.

It is accepted that either reduced perfusion of the brain or hypoxia, or both of these, precede anaerobic metabolism (and thus acidosis) leading to irreversible neuronal damage. The early stages of this process are reversible. (Anthony and Levene, 1990). Signs of hypoxia during labour pose several problems. It is difficult to know whether the fetus is successfully adapting to stress or is beyond its limits of compensation. These adaptations include episodes of anaerobic metabolism and maintaining blood flow to vital organs (Anthony and Levene, 1990). Such adaptations give rise to acidosis. It is not possible to determine form a single pH value whether or not the fetus is temporarily acidotic and is compensating or seriously distressed. It is thought that abnormalities of the fetal heart rate may be related to acidosis. It has been found that less than two per cent of babies with a normal fetal heart rate trace are acidotic, however only about 50 per cent of babies with severely abnormal traces have significant acidosis (Beard et al, 1971). EFM then is a poor indicator of the acidotic state of the fetus.

Asphyxia at birth is then a poor indicator of long-term neurological damage. One of the best ways of identifying the risk of long-term morbidity is the detection of abnormal neurological signs which indicate hypoxic ischaemic encephalopathy (HIE) (Hull and Dodd, 1991). HIE is characterized by a collection of signs seen in the first hours and days of life, including feeding abilities, level of consciousness, seizures and the need for ventilatory support.

Uterine contractions

Uterine contractions can indirectly influence the fetal heart rate by inhibiting blood flow to the fetus. Uterine contractions are crucial to labour. They have to be effective and efficient to expel the fetus. A well grown baby tolerates this stress readily. It is the growth retarded and preterm babies with little glycogen reserve that are susceptible to the changes in maternal uterine blood flow as a result of contractions.

Uterine contractions increase myometrial pressure, which can hinder placental flow by compressing the branches of the uterine arteries found in the myometrium (Ramsey, Corner and Donner, 1963). Therefore, uterine contractions can decrease the rate of maternal blood flow to the placental site. The amount the maternal blood flow decreased depends on the frequency, intensity and duration of the contractions. Thus uterine contractions represent a potential hypoxic event. Normally the uterine contractions are well within the compensatory capabilities of the fetus. It is still important however to ensure that the uterus relaxes between contractions to allow adequate perfusion (Whittle, 1988).

KEY FACTS

- Cardiac function is dependent on adequate oxygenation and oxygen transport.

- Oxygen transport is impossible without cardiac output.

- The initial response to oxygen deprivation is to increase gradually the baseline fetal heart rate in reaction to sympathetic activity.

- With continued oxygen deprivation fetal blood pressure rises.

- A rise in blood pressure results in parasympathetic stimuli and a decrease in the fetal heart rate.

- Inadequate oxygenation leads to the anaerobic metabolism of glycogen and acidosis which adversely affects cardiac function.

- The ability of the fetus to compensate for hypoxia is dependent on several factors. Its reserves of glycogen, gestational age, well-being, previous experience of hypoxic events, the length of time and severity of the hypoxic episode.

- The relationship between fetal hypoxia, asphyxia at birth and cerebral palsy is not known.

- Uterine contractions are a potential hypoxic event.

CHAPTER THREE

The Practicalities of Electronic Fetal Heart Rate Monitoring

Electrocardiotocographs have become extremely sophisticated. However, there are some fundamental principles for obtaining a trace of good quality. EFM is only of value if the person observing the machine is familiar with how it works and is able to interpret the tracing so that the appropriate action can be taken. As with all aspects of midwifery it is important that the midwife is thoroughly conversant with normal traces for the fetal heart and uterine activity.

This chapter covers the following:

- the principles which ensure a high quality trace
- the use of telemetry
- Computer analysis of fetal heart rate patterns
- a review of uterine activity in relation to electronic monitoring
- the normal fetal chart rate trace:
  - its characteristics
  - variability
  - beat to beat variation
  - sleep periods
  - accelerations
- checklist for describing or examining a cardiotocograph tracing
- troubleshooting

Getting a good trace

Prior to the commencement of continuous fetal monitoring, the midwife needs to prepare the woman in a similar way to that detailed earlier for intermittent auscultation.

- The woman needs to be aware of what is going to be done, and why, and made comfortable. She will need to remain reasonably still if external transducers are being used, and in some instances the woman's comfort should be weighed up against the need to monitor the fetal heart continuously. Frequent change of positions may necessitate repositioning of the transducers. Prior to the commencement of monitoring the midwife needs to encourage the woman to empty her bladder and subsequently give her the opportunity to do so at two-hourly intervals.

- The transducer to record the fetal heart rate and uterine activity may only be placed correctly after the midwife has carried out a detailed abdominal palpation.

- The midwife needs to ensure that the cardiotocograph is connected properly, with the transducers plugged into the appropriate connectors and the power cord into the electric socket. The ultrasound transducer can be checked by gently touching its underside to produce a sound similar to a microphone being lightly tapped. Aqueous gel needs to be applied to the ultrasound transducer to aid transmission of the ultrasound waves. If this transducer is not properly applied artefacts may appear which can be confused with abnormal fetal heart patterns particularly decelerations. The belts which hold the transducers in place need to be tightened so they do not slip, causing the signal to be lost.

- If the woman is obese the thickness of the abdominal wall may make obtaining a good trace difficult. If it is imperative that the fetal heart is continuously monitored during labour the midwife may consider applying a fetal scalp electrode.

- Care should be taken to avoid contamination both of the fetus and medical attendants. However, the midwife needs to be mindful of her own area's HIV policy which may state that application of a fetal scalp electrode is contraindicated in high-risk women and those who are seropositive.

- Very frequent fetal movements may make a trace difficult to obtain, so it may be more appropriate for the midwife to delay performing the trace until the fetus is less active.

- The strength of the contractions can only be estimated using the external transducer, but the tension of the belt affects the recording of the contraction strength, so manual palpation of contractions to assess their strength needs to be performed by the midwife periodically. (Some monitors use beltless tocotransducers applied to the abdomen using disposable adhesive base plates.)

The use of telemetry

Women and their partners are now requesting a more personal and humanized birth experience. The use of EFM can detract from this experience. The presence of a fetal monitor in a birthing room can be quite intrusive as it is accompanied by wires and mechanical sounds and restriction of movement. Most women will feel more comfortable during labour if they are able to move as they wish and subsequently are less likely to require as much pain relief (Milner,1986; Odent,1984).

However, as previously discussed it may be important that the fetal heart is continuously monitored. The use of telemetry helps women to remain mobile without the loss of continuous EFM. Telemetry uses radio waves so that the fetal heart beats and the uterine contractions can be recorded by remote control. The woman wears a transducer either by a shoulder strap or other device and then the signals from the fetal heart rate and the uterine contractions are continuously transmitted to a receiver which is connected to the fetal monitor. The fetal heart rate and the uterine activity are printed on to the graph paper after the monitor has processed the information. It is also possible for the midwives' station to have a central monitor display where tracings from several mothers can be displayed.

Telemetry can also be set up in a mother's own home antenatally where the data can be transmitted via a modem to the receiver unit which is connected to a printer which produces the graph of the fetal heart trace and the uterine contractions.

Computer analysis of fetal heart rate patterns

In an attempt to eradicate the problems of trace interpretation, computer analysis of fetal heart rate patterns have been investigated and developed (Dawes et al 1992; Uzan, Fouillot and Sureau 1991). However the computer programmes are dependent on the current knowledge of fetal heart rate patterns which have not been found to correlate well with long-term outcome (Grant et al, 1989; Rosen and Dickinson, 1993). The use of computer analysis of fetal heart rate patterns has to be considered very carefully because of the risk of even more loss of contact between mother and midwife.

Uterine activity

Uterine contractions provide valuable information about the progress of labour. In order to assess contractions clinically a hand is placed lightly on the abdomen over the fundal region of the uterus. The resting tone of the uterus is between 4 and 10 mmHg. During labour the resting tone of the uterus needs to be low so that placental circulation is resumed between contractions to reduce the risk of fetal hypoxia. The woman does not usually feel the pain of the contraction until it reaches 20 mmHg.

As the intensity of the contraction builds up the fundus and the rest of the uterus becomes hard – this can be felt by the palpating hand. The intensity of the contractions is crudely reported as mild, moderate or strong in nature. The duration of the contraction can be timed whilst the palpating hand gently rests on the fundal region. The frequency of the contractions is assessed by timing the interval from the onset of one contraction to the onset of the next.

Uterine activity can be electronically recorded antenatally and during labour. The fetal heart is monitored at the same time to assess how the fetus is coping with any uterine activity if present. However, Olah et al (1993) propose that although palpation and recording of contractions can give an indication that normal labour is progressing, research can be cited that questions whether this is so when oxytocin is used. External contraction transducers can only accurately record the frequency of the contractions. An intrauterine pressure catheter can be inserted internally, although its use is not widespread (Gibb,1993). Indeed, randomized controlled research trials have not demonstrated that using an internal intrauterine catheter is superior to external methods of contraction assessment (Olah et al (1993). The obese woman, however, presents particular problems for assessment of contractions both by external palpation and internal monitoring using an intrauterine catheter.

Care of the monitor

Equipment for electronically monitoring the fetal heart is expensive. Monitors for intrapartum use can cost in the region of £8,000 and are, therefore, valuable pieces of equipment. It is expected that they will be used exhaustively and have been designed so that they can be used 24 hours a day, seven days a week. Nevertheless, people who use the machines need to know how to use them correctly so that any faults that may arise are not user-related. All machines will be accompanied by instructions and all users should read these carefully. In-service training should also be provided so that all staff are familiar with the machines used in their own unit. The machines should also be regularly checked and maintained so they are kept in good working order. (See Appendix I for a checklist which can be used to ensure a good quality trace.)

The normal fetal heart rate trace

Characteristics

The normal fetal heart rate trace has the following characteristics:

- A fetal heart rate of 110–50 bpm (International Federation of gynaecology and Obstetrics (FIGO),1987). (It is slightly higher in the preterm infant, for example it may be 160 bpm in the 20 week fetus (Tucker,1992)). As the fetus matures so does the parasympathetic nervous system and the baseline fetal heart rate decreases. The baseline fetal heart rate is defined as the heart rate when there is no stimulation or stress to the fetus such as in labour.

- A baseline variability of between 5-10 beats per minute.

- Reactivity to stimulation, for example, fetal movements, contractions.

- No decelerations.

Let us examine two of the above terms namely *baseline fetal heart rate* and *variability of the baseline*.

The baseline fetal heart rate is the rate which is present:

(a)   when the woman is not in labour
(b)   when the fetus is not moving
(c)   during the interval between labour contraction
(d)   when the fetus is not being stimulated, for example, during a vaginal examination or application of a fetal scalp electrode
(e)   the majority of time between any accelerations or decelerations.

A *reactive trace* is indicative of fetal well-being. A trace is said to be reactive if a normal baseline rate, normal baseline variability and accelerations are observed. The baseline fetal heart rate is assessed by observing the fetal heart rate for a ten-minute period. The range of the fetal heart rate is the maximum and minimum rate achieved during 80 per cent of the observation period, for example 140–152 bpm. (This is, of

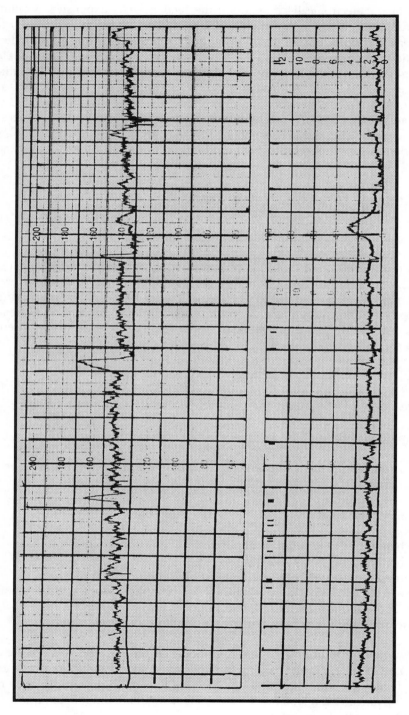

Fig. 3.1: Example of a normal trace

course, easier to state in theory than to achieve in practice.) A trace is termed *reactive* if two accelerations can be observed in a 20-minute trace.

If there has been a change in the range for more than ten minutes a new baseline rate is said to have been established. Changes which persist for less than ten minutes are called transient elevations (Gibb and Arulkumaran, 1992).

Variability of the baseline heart rate

This is the normal irregularity of the fetal heart which is shown as an oscillating pattern demonstrating frequent changes in the fetal heart rate. The common use of the term 'beat to beat' variation is misleading. Each beat of the fetal heart can only be recorded by electrocardiogram (ECG) which is able to record the QRS complex (Dawes, 1993). Therefore, CTG machines give an average rate over a number of beats (the beats will depend upon the make of machine). Thus, a trace obtained through methods other than an ECG is not recording beat to beat variation.

A normal baseline variability is greater than 11 beats per minute but less than 25 beats per minute (Gibb and Arulkumaran, 1992). Variability may be short- or long-term.

Short-term variability is where there is a change in the fetal heart rate from one beat to the next. Long-term variability is where the fetal heart rate fluctuates by 3–5 cycles per minute. Therefore, variability may be decreased or increased. This is difficult to identify on traces which have been recorded using a paper speed of less than 3cms per minute so an averaging technique is used (Gibb and Arulkumaran, 1992).

It should be remembered when examining American texts that the traces will appear quite different in comparison to European texts because different paper speeds and scales are used (Freeman, Gorite, Nageotte, 1991).

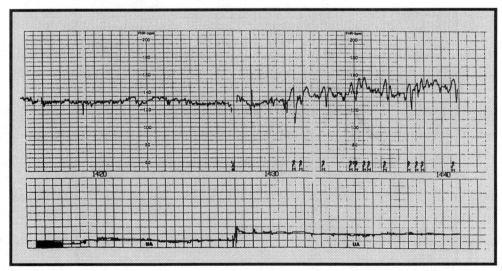

Fig. 3.2: Fetal sleep trace later with acceleration and periodic acceleration and movement, short-and long-term variability

Fetal sleep

A non-reactive trace due to fetal sleep will usually be normal if repeated later (Spencer,1992). If the fetal sleep lasts longer than 20–30 minutes decreased long-term variability is evident.

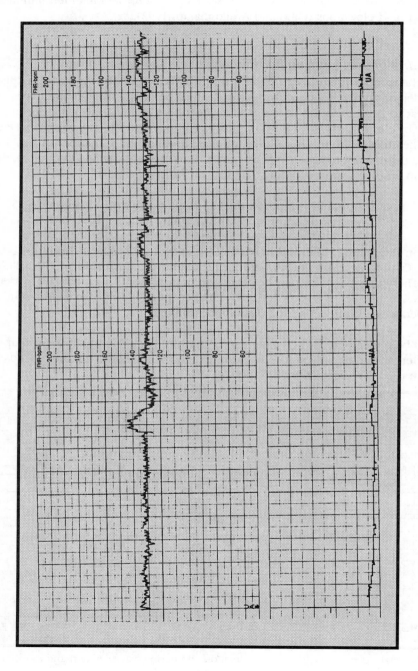

Fig. 3.3: Example of a fetal sleep trace

Accelerations

Accelerations are transitory increases of at least 15 bpm above the baseline rate and lasting for at least 15 seconds (Eganhouse and Burnside, 1992). Accelerations in the fetal heart rate together with good variability is indicative of the fetus having an active phase. Accelerations of the fetal heart indicate fetal well-being. They are mostly associated with fetal movement and uterine contractions.

When the fetus is very active many accelerations may be observed. This may be confused with a tachycardia. Other clues will aid interpretation of this trace. The trace is unlikely to be suspicious in a fetus that is the correct size for its gestation, has a normal amniotic fluid volume and moves frequently. 'An hypoxic fetus with a tachycardia with or without decelerations does not move actively.' (Gibb and Arulkumaran, 1992).

However, in some instances it may be difficult to distinguish between frequent accelerations and tachycardia. Further assessment needs to be made in such situations using biophysical assessment if the difficulty presents antenatally, or using fetal blood sampling during labour.

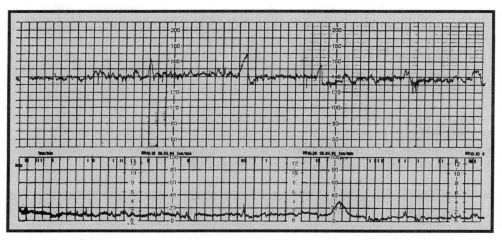

Fig. 3.4: Trace demonstrating a normal baseline FHR and periodic accelerations

Checklist to be considered when describing or examining a cardiotocograph tracing

- Technical quality
- Length of time fetal heart rate was monitored
- Baseline rate
- Baseline variability
- Periodic changes: accelerations and decelerations
- Uterine activity
- Fetal movements

Troubleshooting

Correct interpretation of the trace is important so that the appropriate management action is taken. However, errors may occur in the way a fetal heart rate tracing is performed which may make it misleading.

The midwife must be aware of the errors that can occur in the way the fetal heart tracing is recorded and take steps to avoid this eventuality. Errors may be due to the following:

- A poor signal which makes the tracing of poor quality and difficult to interpret.
- Failure to record the contractions – this makes it impossible to interpret the significance in the altered heart rate pattern.
- Recording of the maternal heart rate instead of the fetal one.
- Failure to record all significant information on the graph paper.
- Failure to check paper speed prior to interpretation of the trace. A speed of 3cm/minute will look quite different from 1 cm/minute. Paper speed can be adjusted on most modern fetal monitors. They are usually set to deliver the paper at 1cm/min.
- Poor contact between fetal scalp electrode and the fetal scalp, which may necessitate reapplication or use of the external ultrasound transducer. The plate on the mother's thigh must be checked to ensure proper application.
- Using transcutaneous nerve stimulation (TENS) for pain relief in labour. This can cause artefacts to appear on the tracing. If TENS is being used and EFM is required the ultrasound transducer should be used.

KEY POINTS

- In order to interpret a fetal heart trace appropriately it needs to be acknowledged that the fetus can have active and quiet periods.

- During active periods the fetal heart trace shows good variability and accelerations.

- During quiet sleep periods there is decreased long-term variability in the fetal heart rate which can last up to 40 minutes.

- A normal antenatal trace has a baseline 110–150 bpm; range of baseline variability 5–25 bpm; no decelerations except occasional, mild and of short duration; and the presence of two or more accelerations during a ten-minute period (FIGO,1987).

- A normal intrapartum trace should have a baseline rate of 120–150 bpm, baseline variability 5–25 bpm, no decelerations.

- The midwife needs to prepare the woman and pay attention to correct use of the equipment – this will help in gaining a good trace.

- If EFM is essential but the woman wishes to remain mobile, the use of telemetry will make the equipment less restrictive.

- Electronic fetal monitors are valuable pieces of equipment and need to be regularly checked and maintained so they are kept in good working order.

- The use of computer analysis of fetal heart rate patterns has the potential for even more loss of contact between the mother and the midwife.

CHAPTER FOUR

Suspicious and Pathological Fetal Heart Rate Traces

The rationale of EFM is based on the hypothesis that the fetal heart pattern changes in response to hypoxia (Hon, 1968; Itskovitz et al, 1982). However, the relationship of such patterns has not correlated well with neonatal neurological outcome (Curzen et al, 1984; Ellison et al, 1991). The Royal College of Obstetricians and Gynaecologists arranged a Working Party on cardiotocograph technology in May 1990, where it was considered that:

> 'In the absence of an acute event, demise of the fetus is usually (but not invariably) preceded by a pathological fetal heart rate pattern.' (Working Party on Cardiotocograph Technology, 1993).

It has been suggested that only about a third of abnormal CTG traces results in a baby with evidence of asphyxia (Capsticks Solicitors, 1994). If therefore, every abnormal CTG trace was acted upon, a large number of caesareans would be performed unnecessarily. However, 17 per cent of severely asphyxiated babies have had a normal CTG trace throughout labour (Capsticks Solicitors, 1994).

The International Federation of Gynaecology and Obstetrics in 1987 classified fetal heart rate patterns which have been internationally accepted (FIGO, 1987). These definitions of fetal heart rate patterns fall into three broad categories; those concerned with the baseline rate, those concerned with the baseline variability and those that are periodic changes. Once these patterns have been identified they can be interpreted to have three possible meanings:

1. Normal – showing good signs of reactivity and no evidence of hypoxia.
2. Suspicious – showing no reassuring signs but no definite signs of hypoxia either.
3. Pathological – showing definite signs of hypoxia.
(Adapted from FIGO, 1987)

There are also subtle differences in the normal fetal heart rate trace of a preterm fetus compared to that of a full-term. What could be mistaken for a suspicious trace could merely indicate immaturity. This chapter therefore considers the following fetal heart rate patterns:

- Baseline rates: tachycardia and bradycardia.
- Periodic changes: accelerations – shouldering and overshooting; decelerations – early, late and variable.
- Baseline variability: long-term, short-term, sinusoidal and saltatory.
- Preterm patterns.
- Midwifes role

Baseline rates

Tachycardia

Baseline tachycardia is defined as a fetal heart rate of 150 bpm or more in a fetus at term. It is described as moderate if it is between 150–170 bpm, and severe if it is greater than 170 bpm. Moderate uncomplicated tachycardia with good variability is not ominous, especially if the fetus is preterm. However, baseline tachycardia accompanied by other high-risk factors, such as reduced fetal movements, decreased variability and/or decelerations, however shallow, needs to be considered very carefully and may be indicative of hypoxia (FIGO, 1987).

Baseline tachycardia can be due to:

- preterm gestation
- developing hypoxia
- maternal anxiety and maternal pain
- maternal dehydration
- fetal activity
- fetal infection and pyrexia
- maternal infection
- maternal hyperthyroidism
- drugs, e.g. atropine, ritrodine
- fetal cardiac anomalies

(Saling and Schneider 1967; Ron et al 1980.)

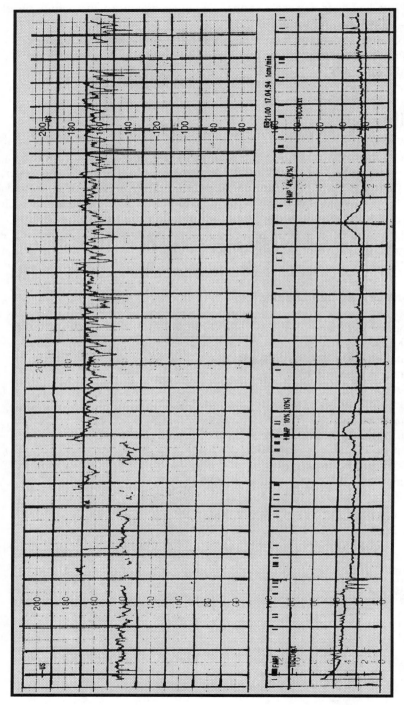

Fig. 4.1: Example of baseline tachycardia

Baseline bradycardia

Baseline bradycardia is defined as a fetal heart rate of 110 bpm or below. It is pathological if it is below 100 bpm (FIGO, 1987). A bradycardia below 80 bpm does not provide sufficient cardiac output, and will result in asphyxia unless it corrects itself or prompt action is taken (Wood and Dobbie, 1989). Mild baseline bradycardia with good variability is not an ominous sign especially if the fetus is mature. However, when baseline bradycardia is accompanied by other high-risk factors the implications can be serious.

Baseline bradycardia can be due to:

• Hypoxia
• Drugs e.g. anaesthetics, analgesics, oxytocin
• Maternal hypotension
• Cord prolapse
• Fetal cardiac anomalies
(Hon, 1968; Calderyo-Barcia et al, 1966.)

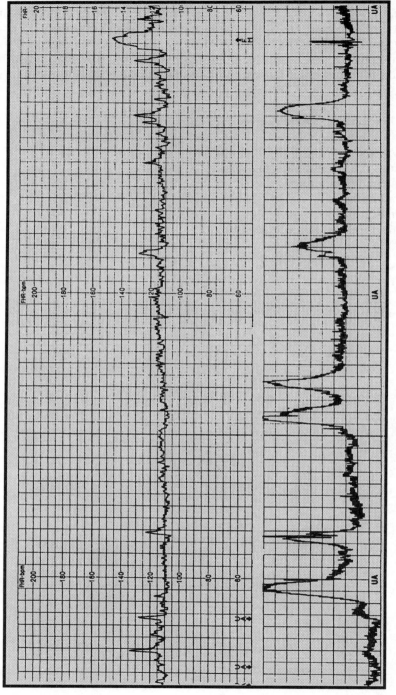

Fig. 4.2: Example of baseline bradycardia

Periodic changes

Accelerations

Accelerations are sometimes associated with variable decelerations. Accelerations can occur immediately before a deceleration: a phenomenon which is known as *shouldering* (James et al, 1976). Shouldering is thought to demonstrate that the fetus is successfully compensating for the effects of cord compression.

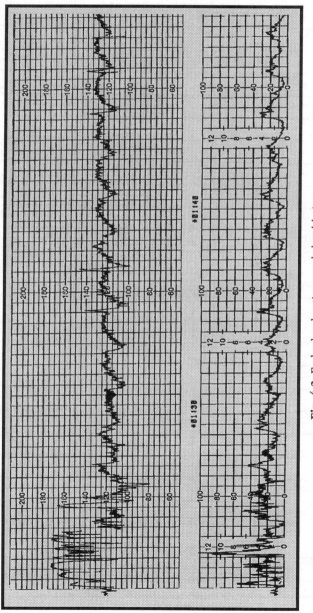

Fig. 4.3: Early decelerations and shouldering

Accelerations which occur immediately after a deceleration are known as *overshooting* (Goodlin and Lowe, 1974).

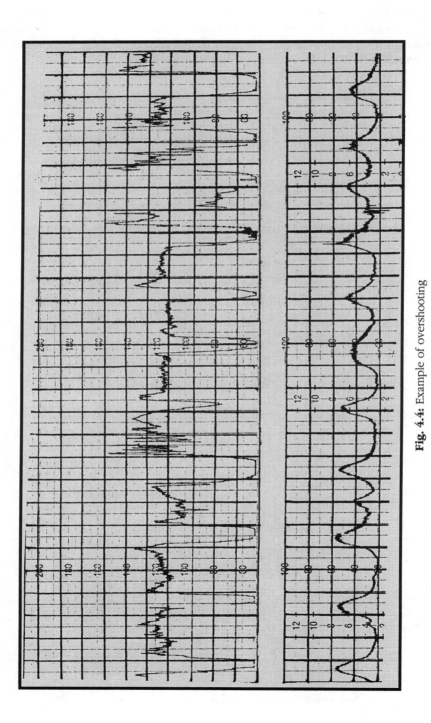

Fig. 4.4: Example of overshooting

Alternatively shouldering and overshooting can occur together, that is immediately before and immediately following the same contraction.

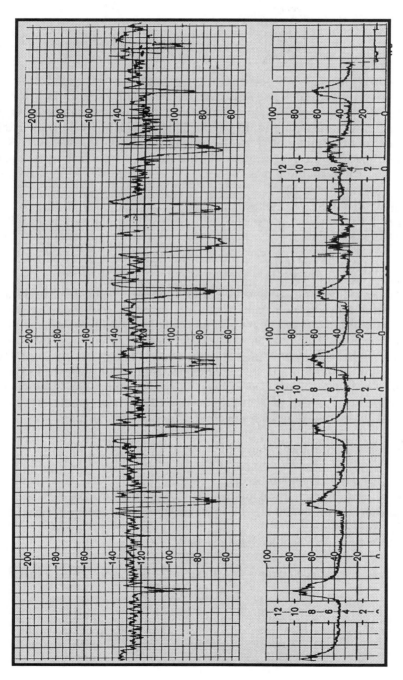

Fig. 4.5: Example of shouldering and overshooting

Overshooting when *not* accompanied by shouldering is an ominous sign indicating hypoxia. Overshooting is suggestive of hypoxia when the fetal heart rate takes longer to return to the baseline (giving a rounded shape to the trace of the acceleration). Overshooting without accompanying shouldering is especially worrying if there is also a decrease in baseline variability.

Decelerations

A deceleration is the temporary decrease of 15 bpm or more below the baseline which lasts 15 seconds or more (Gibb and Arulkumaran, 1992). However, decelerations which decrease less that 15 bpm can be highly significant if there is a loss of baseline variability (Druzin et al, 1979; Modanlou et al, 1977; Hon, 1968). A single deceleration in the fetal heart rate may not be significant. It may be related to a specific episode such as supine hypotension. Provided the fetal heart returns to a normal pattern quickly it requires no specific action. There are three types:

1.   early decelerations
2.   late decelerations
3.   variable decelerations

EARLY DECELERATIONS

Early decelerations occur in conjunction with a uterine contraction in labour, or a Braxton Hicks contraction antenatally. They are a mirror image of the contraction. The lowest point (nadir) of the deceleration should be in proportion to the strength of the contraction. The onset of the early deceleration occurs at the beginning of the contraction and the return to baseline is prompt, before the end of the contraction. The CTG trace of an early deceleration is V-shaped. Early decelerations are usually associated with stimulation of the vagus nerve due to head or cord compression. They commonly occur when the cervix is 4–8 cm dilated, as the head descends. Sometimes they appear in the second stage coinciding with the effort of the mother pushing.

Early decelerations can be worrying if they occur:

* when the woman is not in labour;
* in very early labour, before the head has descended into the pelvis;
* in conjunction with other non-reassuring CTG patterns (complex trace) e.g. loss of baseline variability.

(Hon, 1968; Caldeyro-Barcia, 1966; Hammacherk, 1969)

Repetitive deep early decelerations need careful observation as they may lead to acidosis.

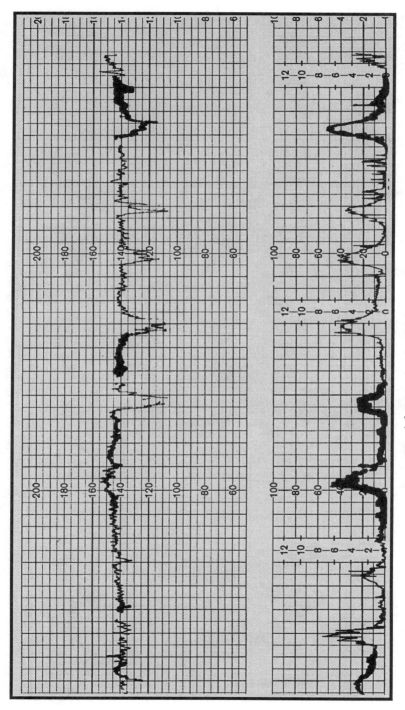

Fig. 4.6: Example of early decelerations

33

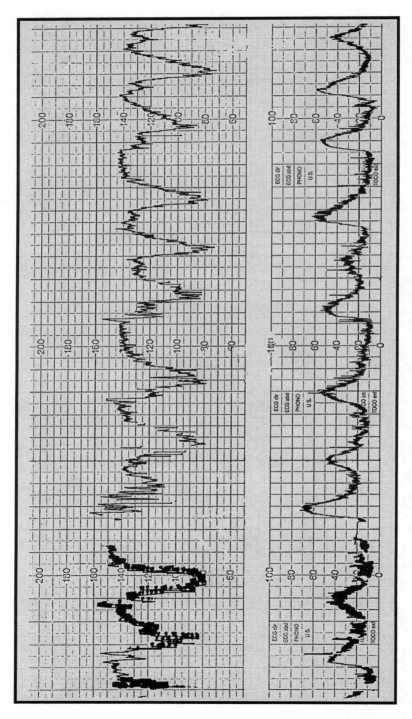

Fig. 4.7: Example of late decelerations

LATE DECELERATIONS

Late decelerations occur after the onset of the contraction. The greater the time lag after the onset of the contraction before the deceleration occurs the more sinister the trace. The depth of the nadir of the late deceleration has little to do with severity, it is the regularity and duration of the deceleration that gives rise to concern.

Late decelerations are associated with:

- maternal hypotension
- excessive uterine action
- inhibition of placental/fetal blood flow

Late decelerations are very ominous if:

- they occur with every contraction;
- there is only a short interval between decelerations;
- they are accompanied by decreased variability (no matter how shallow the nadir);
- the recovery to normal baseline is slow giving a U-shape to the CTG trace.

Prolonged deceleration of the fetal heart rate for two and a half minutes or more which is not related to a contraction is very ominous and indicate bradycardia rather than a deceleration (Hon, 1968; Caldeyro-Barcia, 1966; Hammacherk, 1969).

VARIABLE DECELERATIONS

Variable decelerations are not consistently late or early. They do not have a consistent pattern and vary in onset. Variable decelerations have an irregular shaped CTG trace and are variable in the amplitude of the nadir. Variable decelerations which decrease to a slow rate and last longer and which are slow to recover are an ominous sign, especially if complicated by other abnormal patterns, e.g. a decrease in baseline variability.

Variable decelerations are associated with hypoxia due to:

- cord entanglement;
- cord knots;
- cord prolapse.

(Hon, 1968; Krebs, Petres and Dunn, 1983)

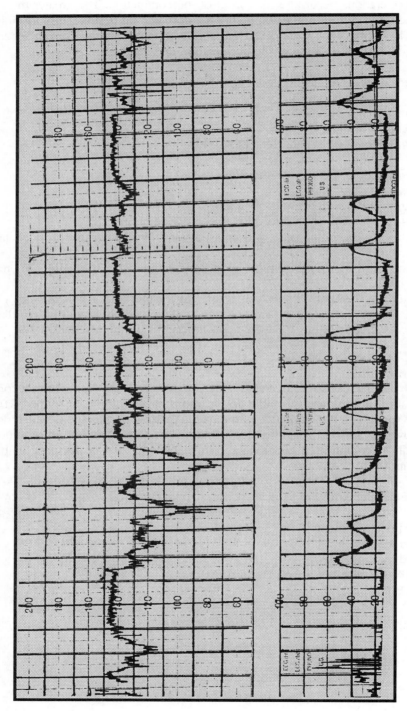

Fig. 4.8: Example of variable decelerations

Baseline variability

The variation of the baseline fetal heart rate between each beat is normally between 5 and 10 bpm. Over the course of one minute, however, there are further rhythmical variations around the baseline. Normally the fetal heart rate varies over a minute, from 15 to 20 bpm. The presence of variability demonstrates the integrity of the fetal nervous system. A reduction in this variation is called a loss of baseline variability and is associated with hypoxia, maternal drugs and cardiac anomalies. Loss of baseline variability is often accompanied by fetal tachycardia and is worrying.

There are two types of baseline variability which can be reduced:

- long-term variability (LTV)
- short-term variability (STV)

When there is loss of both short- and long-term variability the trace has a characteristic flat appearance with little or no variation. A flat trace where there is no variation is very worrying and is a sign of severe hypoxia. Especially ominous is a flat trace with decelerations however shallow (Druzin et al, 1979; Modanlou et al, 1977; Hon, 1968).

Loss of long term variability

When there is a loss in the long term variability (LTV) the beat variation change continues to occur in the short-term between 5 and 10 bpm. This means that the rapid changes that occur around the baseline remain, but the longer term rhythmical variations of the baseline between 15 and 20 bpm over a minute are lost. It is the loss of LTV that is usually seen during the sleep cycles of the fetus, with return to normal reactivity after 30 minutes or so.

Loss of short-term variability

When there is a loss of short-term variability (STV) the rhythmic variations around the baseline of 15–20 bpm over a minute remain, but the rapid changes in the short-term baseline rate of between 5 and 10 bpm is lost. When there is a loss of STV for any significant length of time it is a very ominous sign. It appears as a smooth regular wave on the CTG race and may be continuous or have intermittent runs with oscillations 2–5 times per minute and an amplitude of 5–10 bpm.

Sinusoidal

If the loss of STV is associated with fetal anaemia (such as occurs with rhesus iso-immunisation) it is known as a *sinusoidal* pattern. It is thought to be a premorbidal sign and has a very poor prognosis with 75 per cent mortality. If the loss of STV is *not* associated with fetal anaemia it is described as pseudosinusoidal. Pseudosinusoidal patterns can occur due to severe asphyxia or administration of specific drugs to the mother, such as Alphaprodine (Shenker, 1973; Modanlou and Freeman, 1982; Young et al 1980).

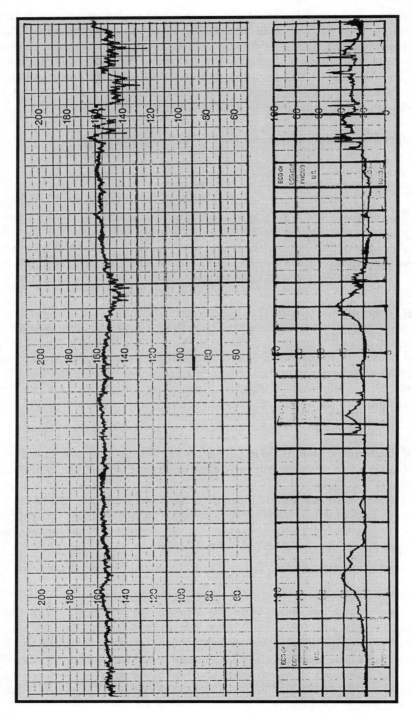

Fig. 4.9: Example of loss of long term variability (LTV)

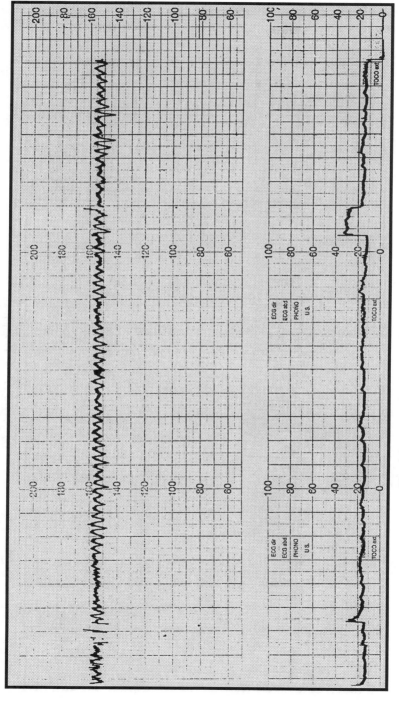

Fig. 4.10: Example of loss of short term variability (STV)

Saltatory

A saltatory pattern is one where there is excessive baseline variability of 25 bpm or greater. The significance of a saltatory pattern is not yet known but is thought to be an increase adrenergic stimulation in response to hypoxia (Druzin et al, 1979; Parer, 1983).

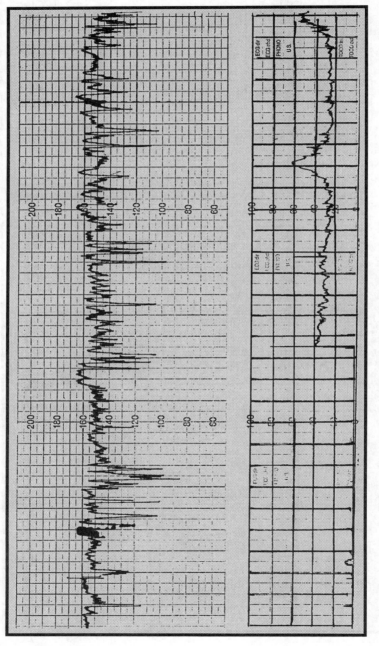

Fig. 4.11: Example of saltatory

Preterm trace patterns

The fetal heart rate pattern is different from that of the full term fetus. The pattern varies as the gestational age of the fetus increases and are quite subtle and complex. A precise and detailed description of preterm fetal heart rate patterns is not possible here but interested readers are referred to Castillo et al (1989) and Eaganhouse and Burnside (1992). Briefly the main differences are that the preterm fetus has a faster baseline rate, different patterns of reactivity and different sleep/activity ratio from the full term fetus. The full-term fetus has a slower baseline rate, increased long-term variability, an increase in the number of accelerations and their amplitude and a different FHR trace in relation to sleep and activity (Castillo et al, 1989; Pillai and James, 1990; Schifrin and Clement, 1990). The changes are indicative of a maturing nervous system.

The baseline fetal heart rate is higher in early pregnancy (about 180 bpm at 15 weeks and 150 at 30 weeks), because the sympathetic nervous system develops earlier in fetal life than the parasympathetic (Walker, 1984). At around 24 weeks gestation, the fetal heart rate will begin to respond to fetal activity. The accelerations of preterm fetuses under 30 weeks gestation tend to be more frequent but do not last as long or increase in rate as much as the more mature fetus. However, decelerations of 10–20 seconds are relatively common in fetuses between 20 and 30 weeks gestation (Pillai and James, 1990). During the second trimester small decelerations may occur in response to fetal movement rather than accelerations (Schifrin and Clement, 1990).

The baseline variability changes in response to the fetal behavioural states of activity and sleep. These differences become more obvious as the fetus matures. There are also subtle differences in the ratio of sleep and activity states of preterm and term fetuses (Eganhouse and Burnside, 1992). This means that what is a normal reactive preterm trace may not have very obvious accelerations, some small decelerations and less baseline variability.

Midwife's role

On identifying a trace the midwife considers to be suspicious or pathological, the midwife needs to continue to closely record the fetal heart and record the maternal vital signs. A senior obstetrician, such as a registrar, should be summoned promptly. The fetal heart rate may improve if the woman's position is altered, e.g. laying on her side or changing sides. In cases where the trace is pathological it is recommended that 100 per cent oxygen is administered to the mother (Freeman, Garite and Nageotte, 1991). If syntocinon is being administered the rate should be reduced or in severely abnormal traces, halted altogether. The accuracy of the electronic recording of the fetal heart rate should be checked by the midwife listening to the fetal heart with a pinnard stethoscope. Liquor should be observed for any signs of meconium staining. The midwife should prepare for a vaginal examination of the woman. A fetal scalp electrode should be applied if the quality of the trace is poor and delivery is not imminent. Fetal blood sampling should be anticipated. Depending on the severity of the trace, the vaginal examination findings and the results of the fetal blood sample, the midwife should be prepared for an emergency surgical delivery, either forceps or caesarean section.

A drop in maternal blood pressure due to an epidural top up can have a profound effect on the fetal heart rate. This is often easily remedied by increasing the administration of intravenous fluids.

Any specific event such as administration of drugs or change of position should be written on the cardiotocographic trace. The midwife must ensure that an accurate continuous trace of the fetal heart rate is maintained. All events and findings should be documented in the records.

The proposed action of the attending obstetrician, or the explanation of why action would not be appropriate, should satisfy the midwife that the woman's best interests are met. If the midwife is not satisfied with the proposed action or inaction she must refer matters to a more senior person until she is satisfied that appropriate care has been given (UKCC, 1989, 1992).

KEY POINTS

- The greater the number of abnormal features present on the trace, the more likely it is to be pathological.

- Good record-keeping is vital for accurate interpretation of the trace and for legal reasons.

- The accuracy of the electronic trace should be checked by auscultation of the fetal heart.

- In the event of a suspicious or pathological trace referral should be made to a senior obstetrician, the woman's position changed, syntocinon reduced or discontinued, her vital signs recorded, the administration of oxygen to the mother considered and a vaginal examination performed. Depending on the well-being of the fetus and the maternal findings, preparation should be made to expedite delivery of the fetus.

CHAPTER FIVE

Intrapartum Case Histories

Introduction

The aim of this chapter is to develop the ability of the midwife to interpret critically cardiotocograph traces. This chapter, therefore, offers the opportunity to consider ten labour case histories in depth. These labour case histories precede the antenatal case histories because the authors felt that antenatal electronic fetal monitoring belongs with the abnormal. A knowledge of normal, suspicious and abnormal traces in labour therefore aids the reader in interpreting antenatal fetal heart rate traces.

The anonymity of the client has been assured and some details changed where necessary. All are interesting in their own right and each raise some very pertinent issues for the care giver particularly in terms of outcome. Each are presented in a similar format and the comments sections at the end are the authors' perspective on the diagnosis and the eventual outcome. These are, of course, the personal viewpoints of the authors.

The literature identifies the fact that interpretation of traces varies from person to person. It is likely, therefore, that not everyone will agree with our interpretation and comments (Lotgeringer et al, 1982; Nielson et al, 1987). We feel that it is the thorough scrutiny of a trace that is important in aiding interpretation. It has taken us a considerable amount of time to describe these short portions of traces. We recognize that we have had the luxury of interpreting them after the event and not in the clinical situation. What is important, nevertheless, is the *process* of interpretation which ensures that a practitioner can account for their actions.

The process used is described in Chapter 3 and comprises the following:

- Technical quality
- Length of time the fetal heart rate was monitored
- Baseline rate
- Baseline variability
- Periodic changes: accelerations and decelerations
- Uterine activity
- Fetal movements

Case study One

A 20-year-old primigravida with no significant medical or obstetric history.

Present pregnancy

Booked at 10 weeks gestation and progressed normally throughout pregnancy until 36 weeks gestation. At this stage diastolic blood pressure was 95 mm/Hg. Clinical examination and ultrasound scan found that the fetal measurements were less than expected for fetal age. She was admitted for observation and rest. Blood pressure remained slightly elevated but stable. Cardiotocograph tracings were performed and were reactive. Ultrasound scan, however, reported cessation of fetal growth. Labour was induced at 39 weeks gestation with prostaglandins, amniotomy and syntocinon. EFM was performed continuously using a fetal scalp electrode.

Labour took some time to become established. An epidural was sited because the woman could not obtain adequate pain relief with pethidine alone. The labour was 6 hours 55 minutes in length although the membranes were ruptured for a total of 11 hours 12 minutes. The woman's blood pressure remained stable throughout labour. Meconium-stained liquor was observed during established labour.

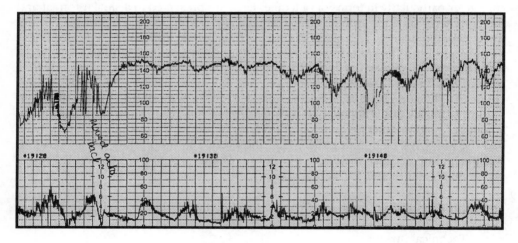

Fig. 5.1: Case study One trace One

Discussion of trace one (Fig. 5.1)

This 10½-minute portion was recorded during the second stage of labour and is of good quality. The second stage of labour had just been confirmed but the woman was not actively pushing. The baseline range is 145–150 bpm. There is some loss of short-term variability. No accelerations are recorded. A number of shallow variable decelerations can be observed. This machine did not have the facility for recording fetal movement. The tocograph indicates that the uterus is contracting 4–5 times in 10 minutes.

This is a worrying trace due to the lack of short-term variability and shallow variable decelerations. Following this episode the woman was turned and remained on her side. The baseline variability and decelerations improved somewhat. The fetal heart pattern continued to be closely observed by continuous monitoring using a fetal scalp electrode. The presenting part was allowed to descend without intervention for the present time.

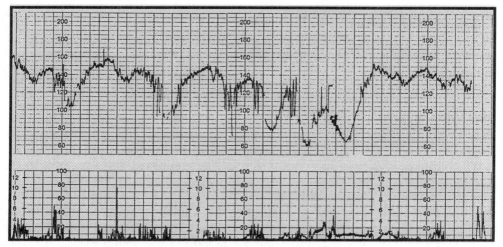

Fig. 5.2: Case study One trace Two

Discussion of trace two (Fig. 5.2)

This section of tracing was recorded 80 minutes later. It is good quality and of 18 minutes duration. The woman was actively pushing at this stage so the uterine activity has been difficult to record. The baseline fetal heart rate is difficult to determine at this time due to numerous decelerations. The baseline variability demonstrates episodes of both poor and good variability. The decelerations appear to be variable but this is difficult to assess retrospectively due to the poor quality of tocographic trace. The impression gained from the trace is that the baseline rate is decreasing as the decelerations become more frequent and are not returning to the predeceleration rate.

Outcome

Due to concerns over the fetal heart rate and maternal exhaustion a forceps delivery was performed. A paediatrician was present for the delivery. A live baby boy was delivered, Apgar scores 7 at 1 minute, 9 at 5 minutes. Oxygen was administered by funnel for two minutes with good effect and suction applied under direct vision. The birth weight was 2.360 kg/5lbs 3ozs. The placenta and membranes appeared healthy.

Comment

This woman required close observation and continuous EFM during labour because of the suspected intrauterine growth retardation and raised blood pressure. Also, syntocinon was used throughout labour and meconium-stained liquor had been observed. The overall clinical picture indicated that an assisted delivery was required. In the event the baby was delivered in a reasonable condition. It is impossible to assess whether this baby would have been delivered in this condition had spontaneous delivery been allowed or whether the intervention prevented further deterioration of the fetal condition.

Case study Two

This woman is a 36-year-old gravida 4 para 3. Her previous pregnancies were all normal culminating in normal deliveries of live babies. She had no medical history of relevance.

Present pregnancy

This woman conceived with a new partner. At 32 weeks gestation the maternal haemoglobin was 10.8g/dl which was successfully treated with oral iron. At 35 weeks gestation spontaneous labour occurred which was not suppressed. She was very anxious and an epidural was sited on her request. As this was a preterm labour EFM was used.

The following trace is the last 28 minutes of the continuous trace recorded before delivery. Similar abnormalities of the fetal heart rate had been observed in the previous hour, therefore, FBS was performed and the blood pH was found to be 7.33. The woman's cervix rapidly progressed to full dilatation following fetal blood sampling.

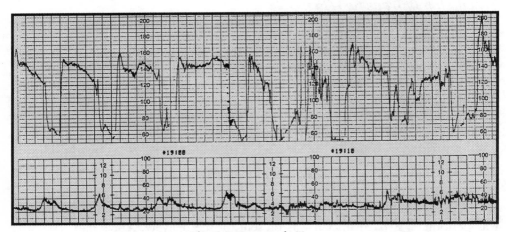

Fig. 5.3: Case study Two

Discussion of trace (Fig. 5.3)

This is a good quality trace, the fetal heart rate being recorded using a fetal scalp electrode. It is difficult to determine the baseline fetal heart rate of this section due to the number of decelerations. There is, however, a portion at 1900hrs which suggests that the baseline rate is between 140 and 150 bpm. The baseline variability is difficult to assess accurately but is suggestive of loss of short-term variability. There are four accelerations following decelerations which could be described as overshooting (an ominous sign when not accompanied by shouldering (Goodlin and Lowe, 1974). There are numerous late decelerations which progressively become more severe and prolonged and give rise for concern. The monitor does not have the facility to record fetal movements. The uterine activity is not clearly demonstrated but difficulties often arise in recording contractions when the mother is actively pushing during the second stage of labour.

Outcome
A normal live female infant was delivered spontaneously after this portion of trace was recorded. Her birthweight was 2.240kg (4lbs 15ozs). The Apgar scores were 9 at 1 minute and 9 at 5 minutes.

Comment
This tracing was highly suggestive of a fetus which was compromised. Despite the ominous signs of the trace the baby was delivered in good condition. However, had spontaneous delivery not been so rapid, intervention would have been justified.

Case study Three
This is the case history of a 28-year-old primigravida woman. She booked at 8+ weeks gestation. She was very anxious and caused concern when she fainted and had a possible epileptic fit whilst having routine booking bloods taken. The woman reported that she had also fainted one month earlier and also at least once a year for some years. She was referred to a neurologist and was reassured that she was not suffering from any neurological condition. Her pregnancy progressed normally until four days after her due date for delivery, when she reported to the antenatal assessment area with a history of only one fetal movement in the previous 24 hours. Her vital signs were normal. A cardiotocograph tracing was performed and a sinusoidal trace was identified. She was transferred immediately to the delivery suite where the fetal heart rate continued to be monitored until an emergency caesarean section was performed two hours after admission.

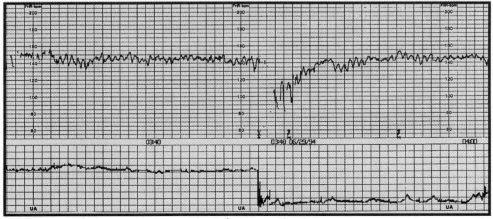

Fig. 5.4: Case study Three

Discussion of trace (Fig. 5.4)

This is a 28 minute section of a continuous fetal heart rate tracing following admission to the antenatal assessment area. The trace is of good quality. The fetal heart was recorded using ultrasound. The baseline fetal heart rate is between 140 and 150 bpm. The undulating appearance of the fetal heart is highly suggestive of sinusoidal rhythm which is associated with fetal anaemia. There are no obvious accelerations, but a significant deceleration dropping to 85 bpm, lasting approximately 1 1/2 minutes. This could possibly be described as a late deceleration. There does appear to be some uterine activity just prior to the deceleration but as the abdominal transducer was recalibrated at this point it is difficult to assess the uterine activity accurately. The woman, however, was not in labour, making this deceleration more significant especially in conjunction with a sinusoidal pattern. Two fetal movements are recorded in this 28 minute period. It may be coincidental that the fetal heart rate began to recover from the deceleration following the fetal movement.

Outcome

A live female infant was delivered by emergency lower segment caesarean section. The cord was around her neck. The Apgar scores were 4 at 1 minute, 7 at 5 minutes and 9 at 10 minutes. Thick meconium-stained liquor was found at delivery. There was no evidence of retroplacental haemorrhage and the placenta was described as healthy. The baby was very pale and was immediately transferred to the neonatal unit. The provisional diagnosis was fetal-maternal haemorrhage. Blood was taken for full blood count, grouping and cultures. The baby's haemoglobin was found to be 4.1g/dl. The plan was to transfuse the baby as soon as possible, closely observe her and keep her warm.

The baby was nursed in an incubator in air and an intravenous infusion was commenced with ten per cent Dextrose prior to 30ml of blood being transfused over 30 minutes followed by a further 48ml over four hours. The father visited and was kept fully informed of the baby's progress. The baby made a good recovery with all observations normal. She was transferred to a cot the next day and was bottle-feeding well. The mother visited the baby and was delighted to find that she was well and could return with her to the ward.

Comment

This was a remarkable case and demonstrates the relevance of maternal anxiety and the reporting of reduced fetal movements. There was no history of maternal blood loss, abdominal pain or any other signs or symptoms to indicate that anything was amiss apart from the history of reduced fetal movements and the abdominal cardiotocograph trace.

Case study Four

A 27-year-old primigravida who had no notably relevant history.

Present pregnancy

She booked at 8+ weeks gestation and the ultrasound scan which was performed at that time confirmed her dates. She progressed normally until she was 33 weeks gestation when, on clinical examination, intrauterine growth retardation was suspected. Measurements of the fetus taken by ultrasound scan suggested a fetus of 30 weeks gestation size. Doppler flow studies were normal and cardiotocograph tracings were reactive. Serial scans showed that fetal growth was slow but progressive and an adequate amount of liquor was present. All other antenatal observations were normal and continued to be carefully monitored.

At 40 weeks gestation this lady went into spontaneous labour which lasted 9 hours 10 minutes. Continuous EFM was performed in response to the intrauterine growth retardation. Four hours 15 minutes later the cervix was assessed as being 4cm dilated and 100mg pethidine was administered intramuscularly for pain relief. The liquor was found to be clear on rupture of membranes.

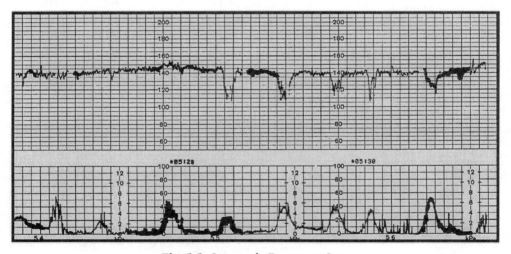

Fig. 5.5: Case study Four trace One

Discussion of trace One (Fig. 5.5)

This is a 26 minute portion of trace recorded during labour. At this time the woman's cervix was 3cm dilated and prior to analgesia being administered. This trace is of reasonable quality but patches of it are blurred due to a technical problem in the recording machinery. The fetal heart was recorded by ultrasound transducer. The baseline rate is between 135 and 145 bpm. There is some loss of long-term variability. There are five early decelerations slowing to around 110 bpm, lasting 30 seconds with no accelerations. The tocograph shows contractions increasing in frequency to about four every ten minutes. The machine did not have the facility to record fetal movements automatically.

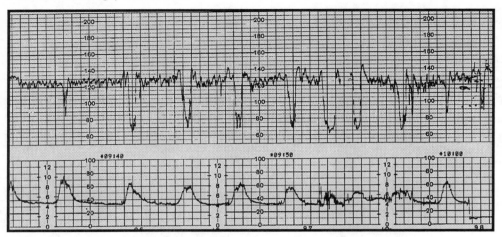

Fig 5.6: Case study Four trace Two

Discussion of trace Two (Fig. 5.6)

This is a 28 minute portion of the continuous labour trace. It was recorded when the cervix was approximately 6cm dilated. It is of good quality. Pethidine had been administered one hour previously. Fetal blood samples were taken shortly afterwards. The baseline fetal heart is between 120 and 130 bpm with good variability. There are numerous early decelerations, several demonstrating both slight shouldering and overshooting. The decelerations are occurring with every contraction and reducing to 80 bpm or more and lasting 30 seconds. Fetal movements are not recorded.

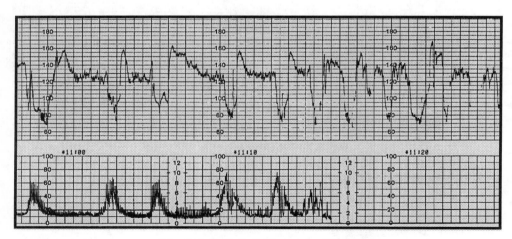

Fig. 5.7: Case study Four trace Three

Discussion of trace Three (Fig. 5.7)

This was recorded during 28 minutes of the second stage of labour. The woman was actively pushing at this time. The fetal blood sample taken one hour previously found a pH of 7.32, which was within normal range. The trace is of good quality. The baseline fetal heart rate is between 125 and 135 bpm with good variability. There are variable decelerations with every contraction. The variable decelerations are dipping down to around 80 bpm and lasting about 45 seconds. This trace demonstrates significant overshooting with the fetal heart accelerating to 155–160 bpm, taking 30 seconds or more to return to the baseline.

Outcome

The woman progressed to a spontaneous vertex delivery of a live female infant with an Apgar score of 9 at one minute and 10 at five minutes. The cord was around the neck, shoulders and leg and a true knot was found in it. The baby's birthweight was 2.285kgs (5lbs 1ozs). Both were transferred home five days after the delivery. The baby was breastfeeding well.

Comment

Despite a very worrying trace the outcome was good. In retrospect it is possible to say that the alterations in the fetal heart rate pattern were the result of cord entanglement and the true knot. However, it is impossible to assess the reason for this except that the fetus was very active, even though growth retardation was suspected and confirmed on birthweight. The use of FBS in this situation avoided an unnecessary lower segment caesarean section. This demonstrates the importance of having FBS facilities when EFM is being used.

Case study Five

A 17-year-old woman who booked at 12 weeks gestation. She had no relevant history.

Present pregnancy

Her pregnancy progressed without any problems. However, she did not go into spontaneous labour. At 42+ weeks gestation she was induced with vaginal prostaglandins, syntocinon infusion and amniotomy. Meconium-stained liquor was found at amniotomy which was described as 'moderate green staining'. She requested an epidural anaesthesia. EFM was indicated on account of the use of oxytocic drugs and the meconium stained liquor.

She progressed quite well and six hours after induction, when her cervix was 3–4cm dilated, occasional early decelerations were noted on the cardiotocograph trace. These decelerations gradually worsened and 8 hours after induction regular variable decelerations were noted. A fetal blood sample was found to be pH 7.3. The variable decelerations continued and a further fetal blood sample was taken two hours after the first which identified a pH of 7.20. At this stage the cervix was 5cm dilated, therefore, an emergency caesarean section was performed 10½ hours after induction.

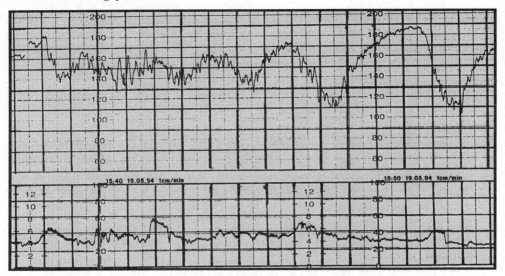

Fig. 5.8: Case study Five

Discussion of trace (Fig. 5.8)

The trace is of good quality. The fetal heart was recorded by fetal scalp electrode. This 18 minute section is part of the continuous trace recorded in labour just prior to the second fetal blood sampling when the woman's cervix was 5cm dilated. An epidural top-up had been administered 45 minutes earlier. It is difficult to determine the baseline rate from this section of the trace. The baseline rate had, however, been between 140 and 150 bpm earlier in the labour. There is good baseline variability. The trace shows late decelerations down to 110 bpm lasting approximately one minute. There is a progressive acceleration rising to 185 bpm. This rise is continuous following a late deceleration and only decreases when the following late deceleration occurs. The uterine activity is not particularly clear but suggests 2–3 contractions every ten minutes.

Outcome

An emergency lower segment caesarean section was performed under a general anaesthetic soon after the illustrated trace. A live female infant was delivered weighing 3.41 kg (7lb 9oz) with an Apgar score of 7 at one minute and 10 at five minutes. On account of the meconium-stained liquor the baby was sucked out under direct vision. There were no postnatal complications and the mother and baby were transferred home on the sixth postnatal day.

Comment

The continued variable decelerations and rebound tachycardia were of significant severity to cause concern. Two fetal blood samples were taken and an emergency lower segment caesarean section was performed when the cervix was 6 cm dilated. Considering the baby's Apgar at one minute, it is possible that the fetal condition was deteriorating, especially as the pH had decreased from 7.3 to 7.2 over two hours. The timing of the caesarean section was optimal ensuring that the baby's condition was not critical at birth. It is impossible to say what would have happened if this woman had not been delivered when she was – the fetal condition may have deteriorated further or may have been capable of compensation. Similarly we might ask, if this labour had progressed rapidly would a live delivery have occurred?

In reviewing this case it must not be forgotten that this woman was at high risk as meconium had been observed in the liquor following artificial rupture of membranes and syntocinon was being used to induce labour at 42+ weeks gestation. These factors in conjunction with the abnormal fetal heart rate pattern of variable decelerations and periods of tachycardia suggest that this fetus was at risk (McNiven, Roch and Wall,1994).

Case study Six

This 21-year-old woman's only obstetric history consisted of evacuation of the uterus for a hydatidiform mole two years previously. She was still being followed up when she became pregnant.

Present pregnancy

Pregnancy progressed normally until 35 weeks gestation when she was admitted following a small bright red loss per vaginum. This resolved without complication and no cause was identified. At 36 weeks gestation she reported reduced fetal movements and a normal reactive cardiotocograph trace recorded a good number of fetal movements. At 38+ weeks gestation she was readmitted in early labour but complained of constant lower abdominal pain. Continuous EFM was indicated because of her antenatal history of bleeding and reduced fetal movements.

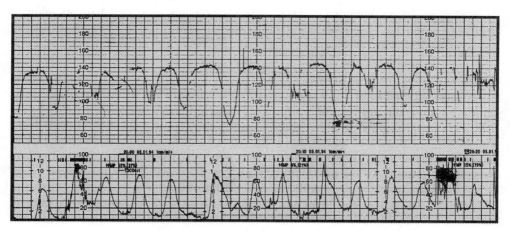

Fig. 5.9: Case study Six

Discussion of trace (Fig. 5.9)

This 20 minute trace is a section of the continuous trace taken during early labour. Immediately prior to this portion of the trace a vaginal examination had been performed and found the cervix to be 3cm dilated. The quality of the trace is good and the fetal heart is recorded by ultrasound. The baseline fetal heart rate is 135–140 bpm. There is loss of short- and long-term variability. There are no accelerations, however, there are numerous late decelerations. The rate to which the fetal heart decreases varies between 70 and 110 bpm lasting 30–45 seconds. The frequency of the uterine contractions is about five every ten minutes. Numerous fetal movements are recorded. This is an ominous trace.

Outcome

An emergency lower segment caesarean section was performed. A live boy was delivered with an Apgar score of 4 at one minute and 7 at five minutes. The baby was resuscitated with suction and oxygen. Birth weight was 2.930 kg (6lb 8oz). The baby was transferred to the neonatal unit for observation. On examination of the placenta a 150ml old blood clot was detected. Cord bloods showed a pH of 6.97. The baby made a good recovery and was transferred to the ward two days following delivery.

Comment

An emergency lower segment caesarean section was indicated on account of the trace demonstrating late decelerations and lack of variability.

Case study Seven

This 27-year-old primigravida booked at ten weeks gestation and had no relevant history of note.

Present pregnancy

All progressed well until the woman was 30 weeks gestation when she complained during an antenatal visit of one episode of 'flashing lights'. Diastolic blood pressure was slightly raised at this time but resolved with rest. At term she spontaneously went into labour. She requested an epidural as the pain of her contractions was not controlled with pethidine alone. The position of the fetus was occipito posterior. She made slow progress in labour so her membranes were ruptured artificially and a syntocinon infusion commenced to augment the labour. EFM was, therefore, indicated. When the cervix was 3cm dilated fetal heart rate decelerations were noted. These were initially early but developed into late decelerations. FBS was performed with normal results. Uterine activity also diminished and no further cervical progress was made.

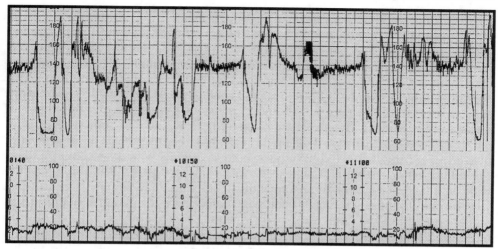

Fig. 5.10: Case study Seven

Discussion of trace (Fig. 5.10)

This is a 28 minute portion of the continuous trace performed during labour. The labour lasted 18 hours and the cervix did not dilate more than 3cm. This section of the trace was recorded approximately one hour prior to delivery by lower segment caesarean section. The trace is of good quality. The fetal heart was recorded by scalp electrode. There are clearly periods of time when the baseline rate is 140–150 bpm. At other times it is difficult to identify the baseline rate due to the varied pattern of the fetal heart rate. Both dramatic accelerations and decelerations can be observed. Where the baseline rate is stable the variability is good. However, the latter part of the trace demonstrates excessive variability. The decelerations are difficult to classify because there is only weak uterine activity. (The uterine activity has in fact diminished from earlier in the labour.) The trace demonstrates the fetal heart rate decreasing to 60–80 bpm and lasting 30–60 seconds. There is a portion where despite intermittent increases in rate the fetal heart rate gradually decreases and could be described as bradycardic, lasting for about ten minutes.

There are several accelerations, some of which are in excess of 40 bpm above the baseline of 140–150 bpm. Several last more than 15 seconds and one acceleration lasts about one minute. All of the accelerations accompany a deceleration.

Outcome

An emergency lower segment caesarean section was performed on account of no progress had been made in labour over a 9 hour period, and because of worsening decelerations of the fetal heart rate pattern. A live female infant in a left occipito position was delivered with an Apgar score of 9 at one minute and 10 at five minutes. The cord was around the shoulder and mouth. Both mother and baby made a good recovery and were transferred home on the fourth postnatal day. The baby was breastfeeding well.

Comment

This woman had been admitted with spontaneous contractions that failed to develop. Labour was augmented but no progress was made. The uterine activity gradually decreased. The fetal heart rate pattern was ominous (decelerations with no contractions) and, therefore, a caesarean section appeared the only option. However, despite the abnormal trace the baby was born in a good condition and was found to quite happy sucking on its cord! This trace was identified as abnormal but it is known that abnormal traces are not particularly reliable indicators of fetal hypoxia. Abnormal traces leave the health professional with a dilemma. Taking action may result in an operative delivery of a baby that could have been born by vaginal delivery without problem. Not taking action, however, could result in having to explain why action was not initiated in the presence of an abnormal trace. Cases are only brought to court when 'experts' have opposing views. If there were consistency of opinion about what was an abnormal trace, no cases would reach court. Either the plaintiff would have to recognize that there was no case to answer or the defendant would settle out of court accepting that the acknowledged abnormality had not been recognized. The trouble with the case (and indeed many others) is not knowing what would have happened if there had been no intervention.

Case study Eight

This is the case history of a 37-year-old woman who was gravida 3 para 2. Her previous pregnancies has been uneventful. The first baby was a boy weighing 2.863 kg (6lb 5oz) and was delivered by Neville Barnes Forceps after a prolonged labour of 20 hours. Her second baby was a girl who weighed 2.892 kg (6lb 61/2oz) who had been delivered normally after a labour of only 2 hours. Following this delivery she had had to have an evacuation for retained products of conception. Both babies had been born with good Apgar scores and were well and breast fed.

Present pregnancy

At booking she was found to have anti-E antibodies. Careful monitoring of titre levels was maintained throughout pregnancy. Her husband was found to be heterozygous for antigen E. The fetus, therefore, had a 50:50 chance of being affected. Serial ultrasound scans identified normal fetal growth.

Pregnancy progressed normally. At 39 weeks gestation she presented with mild contractions and backache. On account of her previous rapid labour she presented herself early. The woman was continuously monitored because of her anti E status. She progressed quite rapidly and reached the second stage of labour within four hours. Worsening decelerations of the fetal heart rate were observed during labour.

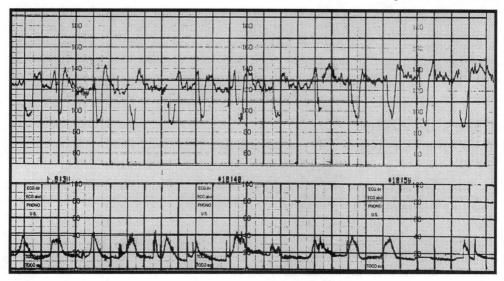

Fig. 5.11: Case study Eight

Discussion of trace (Fig. 5.11)

This is a good quality trace and is an 18 minute section of the continuous trace recorded in labour. It was recorded prior to the vaginal examination which found only an anterior lip of cervix present.

The fetal heart was recorded by fetal scalp electrode. The baseline fetal heart rate is 120–130 bpm. The variability is satisfactory. The decelerations are variable. Although at first glance they appear to be early, careful scrutiny reveals that some of the decelerations are in fact late. The fetal heart rate decreases to between 85–100 bpm and last about 30 seconds.

The pattern of accelerations vary. Some can be seen following the decelerations (overshooting). Others occur prior to the deceleration (shouldering). However, when shouldering is present so too is overshooting. Uterine activity is good with five contractions every 10 minutes and lasting about 30 seconds.

Outcome

This woman delivered a live healthy baby boy weighing 2.880 kg (6lb 2oz) with an Apgar score of 9 at one minute. The labour had been 41/2 hours in total. There was no haemolytic disease of the newborn and mother and baby were transferred home three days after delivery.

Comment

Whilst there are signs of hypoxia this trace suggests that the fetus was compensating nonetheless. When overshooting does occasionally occur on its own it returns to the baseline quite rapidly. It should not be forgotten that labour was known to be advanced (it is easy in retrospect to say all is well). However, had the labour lasted any longer it is impossible to say whether the fetus could have continued to compensate. The ability to predict the outcome based on the fetal heart rate trace alone is exceptionally difficult.

Case study Nine

The following case history is that of a 26-year-old primigravida with no relevant past history.

Present pregnancy

She booked early for midwifery-led care in a consultant unit. There were no problems identified during pregnancy. At 36 weeks gestation she presented with spontaneous rupture of the membranes. Clear liquor was found to be draining per vaginum. She was treated conservatively but did not progress into labour. After 24 hours labour was induced by syntocinon infusion. Labour progressed very slowly. An epidural was sited at the mother's request. The fetal heart rate was monitored electronically because of the use of syntocinon. The fetal heart rate trace pattern was similar throughout labour.

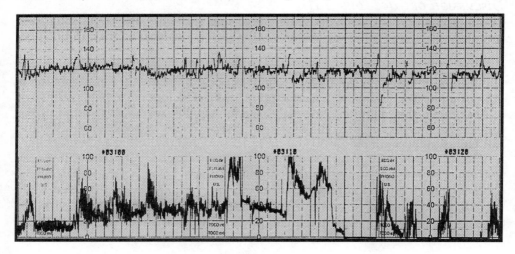

Fig. 5.12: Case study Nine

Discussion of the trace (Fig. 5.12)

The quality of the fetal heart rate trace was questioned in this case. The mother's notes contain a good record of the attempts that were made to ensure an accurate trace was recorded. The machine was changed and the fetal heart rate was recorded by scalp electrode instead of ultrasound. (The rate was checked using a Pinard's stethoscope.) The pattern obtained was always one which could be interpreted as a technical problem with a somewhat tooth-edged appearance.

This is a 28 minute portion of the continuous trace. It is typical of the pattern found during most of the labour. At this time the woman has been in labour following induction for nine hours and one hour later the cervix was found to be fully dilated. An epidural top-up had been administered 20 minutes prior to the trace.

The baseline fetal heart rate is between 110 and 120 bpm. The variability is just about adequate. There are some accelerations rising to 130 bpm lasting about 15 seconds. Two shallow decreases in the fetal heart rate follow a contraction but do not drop more than ten bpm below the baseline rate. They last around 30 seconds. It is difficult to interpret the significance of these fetal heart rate changes. There is one possible deceleration of the fetal heart rate down to 85 bpm but it returns to the baseline rate after about 15 seconds. The uterine activity suggests four contractions every ten minutes.

Outcome

The first stage of labour was ten hours. The second stage of labour was three hours in total but only active for 1½ hours. A ventouse extraction was performed for maternal exhaustion and failure to progress during the second stage of labour. The fetal heart rate never clearly demonstrated a serious problem. A live female infant was delivered with an Apgar score of 3 at one minute and 7 at five minutes. She required resuscitation by ambu bag and mask following delivery. Her birthweight was 2.600kg (5lb 12oz). She was transferred to the ward with her mother and both went home on the third postnatal day.

Comment

This trace is suggestive of lack of variability with significant shallow decelerations. This is, however, stated with the benefit of hindsight and detailed scrutiny. The variability is on the borderline of being normal. There are clearly some changes in baseline rate. In spite of the poor Apgar scores the baby made a rapid recovery following resuscitation. If labour had progressed any longer it is impossible to say whether the outcome would have been any different.

Case study Ten

This is the case history of a 34-year-old woman who was gravida 2 para 0+1. She had suffered a spontaneous abortion at six weeks gestation some 18 months prior to this pregnancy. There was nothing else of relevance in her medical history.

Present pregnancy

She booked early and the pregnancy progressed without antenatal complication. She had booked for midwifery-led care in a consultant unit, but was transferred to consultant care at 42 weeks gestation for induction of labour.

Induction by prostaglandin pessaries, amniotomy and syntocinon infusion. EFM was indicated because of the use of syntocinon. An epidural was sited as pethidine had not been effective. The labour took time to become established. However, once the cervix reached 5cm dilated, rapid progress was made. In total the labour lasted about 12 hours.

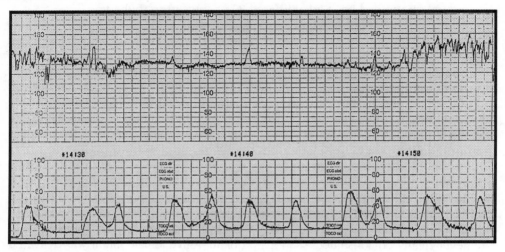

Fig. 5.13: Case study Ten trace One

Discussion of trace One (Fig. 5.13)

This trace was recorded ten hours prior to delivery and two hours following amniotomy. The trace is a 28 minutes section of the continuous trace recorded during labour.

The trace is of good quality. The baseline fetal heart rate is 125–140 bpm. However, the section in the middle illustrates a sleep trace with a baseline 130 bpm with occasional accelerations in response to uterine activity. This is a good example of a fetal heart rate showing a good return to reactivity and variability following a sleep period, indicating the well-being of the fetus.

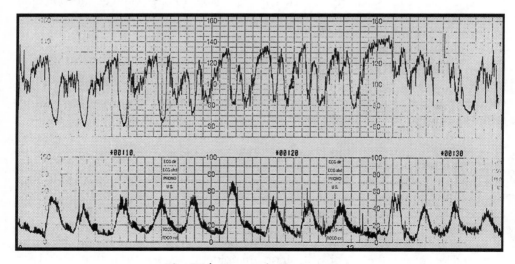

Fig. 5.14: Case study Ten trace Two

Discussion of trace two (Fig. 5.14)

This is a 28 minute section of the continuous trace recorded during labour, recorded during the last hour of labour prior to delivery. As a result of decelerations in the fetal heart rate the syntocinon had been discontinued one hour earlier. The uterine activity continued to be good with five contractions in ten minutes. A fetal blood sample had been taken just after the syntocinon had been discontinued and found the fetal pH to be 7.28.

The baseline had been 125–140 bpm but it is difficult to identify the baseline on this trace because of the frequent changes in the fetal heart rate pattern. Each contraction is accompanied by a variable deceleration. These decrease to between 60–80 bpm and last between 30 and 60 seconds. The variability is good despite the worrying decelerations.

Outcome

On account of this trace the woman was prepared for and delivered by ventouse extraction. A live male baby was delivered and found to have the cord around its body. The baby's Apgar score was 5 at one minute and 9 at five minutes. He required suction and resuscitation by bag and mask but rapidly recovered and was transferred to the ward with the mother. His birthweight was 3.300kg (7lb 5oz). Mother and baby went home on the fourth day following delivery.

Comment

When comparing the two traces the change in the fetal heart pattern can be easily identified. The second trace is suspicious and delivery was expedited. The condition of the baby at delivery indicated that delivery had been required even though he made a good recovery. Syntocinon is a powerful drug and close monitoring of the maternal and fetal condition is required when it is being used. In this case no more than one unit of syntocinon per hour was administered and this was controlled depending on the fetal heart rate response.

CHAPTER SIX

Antenatal Electronic Monitoring of the Fetal Heart

Electronic monitoring of the fetal heart antenatally came about as a result of the experience gained by its use during labour (Cario, 1985). Interpreting fetal heart rate patterns during labour had demonstrated that the stress of contractions can cause a decrease in placental blood flow which could be accompanied by an alteration in the fetal heart rate pattern and potentially cause fetal acidosis. It was natural that researchers should then consider how the stress of labour could be replicated antenatally to identify at-risk pregnancies.

This chapter will consider:

- the indications for using EFM antenatally and the appropriate stage for its use
- the antenatal stress tests
- the use of telemetry antenatally
- the midwife's role and responsibilities in antenatal electronic monitoring of the fetal heart
- some case histories which demonstrate normal and abnormal fetal heart rate patterns.

The use of EFM antenatally

Overview

The search for an antenatal test which can predict fetal morbidity and mortality continues. To date there is still no perfect test. Druzin (1992) in describing antepartum fetal evaluation using continuous EFM states that,

> 'the ability to predict the "healthy fetus" is its strength, the inability to distinguish the "sick fetus" is its weakness' (p.xiii).

What has been observed is that there are characteristic patterns in the fetal heart rate in response to fetal movement. Antenatal stress tests have been developed to try to replicate the stress of labour, gaining insight into how the fetus might fare during labour. The subjective assessment of fetal movement by a woman has long been used as a test for fetal health. Non-stress testing combines maternal perception of fetal movement with recording of fetal heart rate accelerations.

However, one needs to consider the most appropriate stage in pregnancy for using EFM. Devoe (1988) recommends that it is used diagnostically after 30 completed weeks of gestation. Abnormal patterns have been observed in fetuses less than 30 weeks, but because data are scant in extremely preterm fetuses the interpretation of traces at that gestation is problematic. As a result, it is possible to interpret early third trimester traces incorrectly. Therefore, testing, particularly in these instances, must not be used on its own to decide management. (One could argue that this should be predominantly true for all cases.)

The difficult decision to make concerning management when abnormal features of a test are identified is whether to deliver a preterm infant which will require special or neonatal intensive care or await events and allow fetal lung development which may as a result jeopardise the fetus. This decision needs to be made collectively with obstetricians and paediatricians/neonatologists so that all involved are in agreement.

The following antenatal tests are currently being used:

- Non-stress test
- Contraction stress test
- Biophysical profile
- Doppler blood flow studies

The antenatal stress tests

The non-stress test (NST)
The basis of this test is that the reaction of the fetal heart to normal events such as Braxton Hicks contractions or fetal movement is observed. Lee et al (1975) demonstrated that a reactive trace has accelerations and is a good indicator of a healthy fetus. Since then many studies have confirmed that fetal well being can be predicted using a normal reactive non-stress test e.g. Paul and Miller (1978); Evertson et al (1979); Gibbons and Nagle (1980).

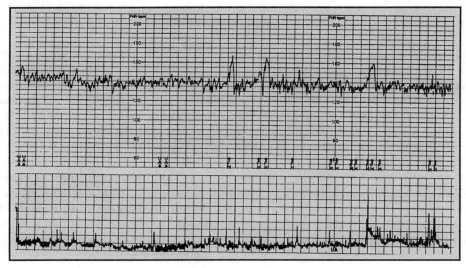

Fig. 6.1: Non-stress test

NST is indicated in high-risk cases where there is potential fetal morbidity and mortality. Examples include:

- Hypertensive disorders
- Diabetes
- Intrauterine growth retardation
- Decreased fetal movements
- Preterm labour
- Twin pregnancy
- Medical conditions e.g. cardiac, renal disease.

Therefore, any disorder which is associated with antenatal and perinatal loss requires increased fetal observation.

Clinicians vary as to how frequently they consider the test should be performed, as each case needs to be individually assessed. Tucker (1992) suggests that for primary surveillance in high-risk cases, such as post maturity, diabetes and intrauterine growth retardation, it could be performed twice weekly. However, where the test is non-reactive, a repeat is necessary within 24 hours or delivery should be expedited.

Mohide and Keirse (1991) express concern about how reproducible the non-stress test is. They cite work which estimates that 10–15 per cent of all records are unsatisfactory. A number of major sources of error have been identified.

First, there appears to be no universal technique for performing non-stress antepartum testing. Each unit decides how long and how frequently to perform the test.

Secondly, appropriate equipment must be used and there must be sufficient expertise to interpret the test's findings, as some equipment may produce errors in the form of artefacts. Interpretation of fetal heart traces continues to be subjective and inconsistent between observers, not only on the same occasion, but also between the same observer on different occasions (Lotgeringer et al, 1982; Nielson et al 1987).

Redman (1993) also argues that scoring systems which have been devised to overcome this problem are difficult to standardize and educating others remains problematic. Therefore, an objective numerical analysis which measures fetal heart rate patterns of interest has been devised. This system (marketed as FM7 System 8000, Oxford Sonicaid) uses a computer with the aim of making the information contained within the fetal heart rate data accessible for interpretation (Redman, 1993). Although the system has been adapted for use in labour, difficulties still persist.

It is stressed, however, that the computer is an aid and is no substitute for clinical judgement which should always have the final say. The system analyses the antenatal fetal heart rate but trials as to its clinical effectiveness have not been completed. The continuing problem is the need to consider the total picture to avoid taking action based on insufficient evidence.

The trace produced may be unsatisfactory because the woman is obese, or because the fetus is active or mobile, or because the fetus is small or preterm.

The gestational age of the fetus needs to be considered because a so-called 'abnormal' fetal heart rate pattern may be described in preterm fetuses.

Fetal rest periods may last for more than 30 minutes and may be confused with a pathological change.

There are many methods used for describing non-stress test results but most include the following:

- baseline fetal heart rate with a minimum amplitude of 10–15 bpm and a minimum duration of 15 seconds
- short- and long-term variability
- active fetal movements and accelerations of the fetal heart rate with spontaneous or stimulated movement
- any decelerations with spontaneous uterine contractions.

Some systems assign scores to the various characteristics. However, the most common method is to assess the trace in terms of whether it is reactive (normal) or non-reactive (abnormal). This assessment is based on the presence or absence of an adequate baseline fetal heart rate, variability and accelerations with fetal movement.

Unfortunately, the non-stress test is not without its problems. Flynn et al (1982) demonstrated that totally different management could be applied in response to identical traces depending on the method used to assess the trace. It has also been reported that obstetricians vary in their interpretation of traces when presented with the same trace on different occasions (Timbas and Keirse, 1978a; Mohide and Keirse, 1991). The non stress test is a relatively good predictor of future events if mortality and morbidity rates are combined. Serial non-stress tests are particularly useful in this respect. However, trials which have evaluated this test recommend that it needs to be supported by other tests which provide additional information in order to manage high-risk cases (Mohide and Keirse,1991).

With the associated difficulties in making a management decision from the information gained from the non-stress test some centres in America still favour the contraction stress test.

Contraction stress test

This test observes features of the fetal heart in the presence of contractions. The reasoning behind this is that a contraction produces a potential hypoxic state for the fetus as intervillous flow may be compromised by compression of the uterine arteries. For the purpose of the test the contractions may be spontaneous or induced, using oxytocin or nipple stimulation. Many centres have discontinued using dilute solutions of oxytocin to induce contractions because they cannot be used in many high-risk cases; such as preterm labour, premature rupture of membranes, placenta praevia,

65

placental abruption (Cario,1985). Also the safety of the test is questionable as there is a risk of hypertonic action which could potentially be accompanied by severe hypoxia and placental abruption.

Mohide and Keirse (1991) discuss the use of nipple stimulation to induce contractions. The mother stimulates her nipples with her fingers or palms or using a warm, moist flannel. This also has many of the disadvantages of the oxytocin-induced contractions and although stimulation can be discontinued, there is a time-lag of more than three minutes from stimulation of the uterus to when the uterine response is greatest. Therefore, Kubli et al (1969) and Hammacher (1969) proposed that the fetal heart rate should be evaluated without inducing contractions.

Other manoeuvres have been described such as abdominal stimulation, and glucose infusions. The use of vibroaccoustic stimulation using an electronic artificial larynx has also been successful in altering the reactivity of the fetus (Smith et al,1986). Devoe (1988) uses five classifications of the contraction stress test:

1. Positive
2. Negative
3. Suspicious
4. Unsatisfactory
5. Hyperstimulation

Unfortunately both antenatal non-stress and contraction stress tests have a high incidence of negative predictive value, i.e. that when they are normal they are excellent predictors of fetal health, but because they both have high false positive results further investigations are required to confirm abnormal findings.

Biophysical profile

Both the non-stress test and the contraction stress test have high false positive rates, therefore, the biophysical profile has been used in an attempt to lower the incidence of unnecessary delivery. The biophysical profile provides more comprehensive information about the fetal condition and any significant observations which increase the risk of fetal death. Manning, Platt and Sipos (1980) describe two types of information which the profile can provide. The profile can make acute observations of fetal heart rate patterns, fetal breathing and body movements, reflex activity and neurologic tone. These features reflect adequate oxygen levels, a normal acid base balance, and sufficient caloric reserves. Also, suggestions of a more chronic state may be observed by assessing amniotic fluid volume and placental grade. This may indicate longer term conditions such as chronic uteroplacental insufficiency. A rating scale is used for each parameter and the test may be approached in different ways.

A non-stress test may be performed first followed by an ultrasound scan in order to make the other observations. Alternatively, EFM and an ultrasound scan may be carried out simultaneously (Devoe,1988). Unfortunately the literature does not establish a standardized test length, although 30–45 minutes is the minimum time needed to allow for fluctuations in fetal activity. Similarly, there is no standardization of maternal condition. Thus for example, decreased fetal movement has been reported when the mother has fasted for a prolonged period (Devoe,1988). This author also suggests that the activity of the fetus is governed by rhythms which occur about once a day. Therefore, in order for the test to be indicative of true fetal state it should be performed at the same time every day. Druzin (1992) reports that there are no contraindications to the test, but that it should be performed at a point in gestation and when the fetus is of appropriate weight for any intervention to provide a reasonable chance of survival.

It may be concluded, therefore, that the non-stress test can be used as a primary screening test, and a contraction stress test and or a biophysical profile augment it in cases where the non-stress test is abnormal. As the preterm fetus is likely to demonstrate a non-reactive non-stress test due to its gestational age, Druzin (1992) recommends that only the biophysical test is performed if the pregnancy is less than 36 weeks gestation. Other potential factors which may affect these screening tests are narcotics and smoking which increase the chance of a non-reactive non-stress test.

Whatever the protocol used for carrying out these observational tests, it is important to integrate the results into the total clinical picture so that decisions concerning management can be made using comprehensive test results and agreement of all clinicians involved in the woman's care.

Doppler assessment of blood flow
As there is still not one ideal antenatal test the search continues for a technique which can prevent fetal morbidity and mortality. Doppler looked extremely promising when it was first used but its place in antenatal screening is still awaiting evaluation through trial results.

Doppler uses an ultrasound beam in which the blood flow in both fetal and placental vessels may be observed. It is non-invasive. The calculation of blood flow velocity is complicated and relies upon the angle which the ultrasound beam adopts. Errors have been reported in the calculations when the angle of the ultrasound beam has been inaccurate. However, it has been found that measurement of the umbilical waveforms is relatively easy to perform and provides reliable information (Druzin, 1992).

There remains a question whether doppler provides superior information to any other test. Although the doppler may provide a normal result, abnormal results may not indicate the need to deliver. As with all other tests, a comprehensive clinical picture needs to be established using a range of diagnostic tools. However, this remains problematic until adequate indicators of long-term outcome are found (Anthony and Levene, 1990).

The use of antenatal telemetry
Dawson et al (1989) discuss how the telephone monitoring systems can be used to reduce the number and duration of hospital admissions for some women with high-risk pregnancies. Women who require electronic fetal monitoring on a regular basis as

part of their antenatal care can have the monitoring performed at home whilst the obstetrician is able to see the graph as it is transmitted via modem to the receiver which is connected to a printer based in the consultant unit. The scheme particularly benefits women who would not normally be admitted but would, nonetheless, benefit from additional observation. The scheme also eliminates the need to visit antenatal day units which provide outpatient electronic fetal monitoring. Dawson et al (1989) report that the scheme has several benefits, not least an economic one. Evaluation found, however, that the scheme was neither more nor less favourable in terms of obstetric outcome, although the women were in favour of it. To date such schemes are not widespread and most units are progressing with antenatal assessment day units as an alternative (Kenyon, 1994).

The midwife's role and responsibilities

Antenatal assessment of fetal well-being is of prime importance for women who are deemed to have high-risk pregnancies. There are still many unanswered questions about fetal outcome and it is hoped that with increased knowledge and improved technology the management of complicated pregnancies will continue to improve. The midwife has a key role in caring for women who undergo the assessments and investigations discussed throughout this chapter. She is in a position to continue to provide individualized care depending upon the woman's needs.

The midwife will be able to aid understanding of any procedures which the woman is subjected to, so that she fully understands the reasons why particular observations are being made and what the eventual outcome might be. The woman will quite naturally be anxious about what is happening and the midwife can play a key role in support and reassurance during the period of investigation. The midwife can explain about the complex machinery to the woman and how it will be applied and what information is likely to be gained about the fetus. Kenyon (1994) believes that this may not prevent the woman from worrying but the support and counselling that the midwife provides may enable the woman and her partner to cope better.

It is also important that in addition to being involved with the procedure itself the midwife needs also to remember to provide basic nursing care, making the woman comfortable and repositioning periodically.

The midwife needs to be vigilant about documenting events and recording any observations made. Prompt reporting of any abnormal events to the medical staff is also important.

The midwife will be extending her skills as a result of her involvement with antenatal investigations and she needs to have had the appropriate training for this role. However, it is important that as a result she does not become deskilled in other aspects of care (Kenyon, 1994).

Antenatal assessment techniques need to viewed as part of the total care of the woman and her partner. Odent (1994) believes that the total health of the pregnant woman needs to be focused upon factors such as her emotional state and her diet. Increasingly more insight is being gained into the long-term effects of the fetus who is compromised in the antenatal period and during labour. The midwife needs to see the individual woman as a holistic ally in the preparation for pregnancy and labour.

Antenatal case histories

The following antenatal histories demonstrate a variety of management issues involved in high-risk antenatal care.

1. Reduced fetal movements at 38 weeks gestation, asymmetrical intrauterine growth retardation
2. Antenatal screening due to previous intrauterine death at 41+ weeks gestation
3. Twin pregnancy
4. Intrauterine death at 30 weeks gestation
5. Intrauterine growth retardation at 38 weeks gestation, maternal malaria.

Case study one

A 29-year-old gravida 2 para 1. EFM formed part of the antenatal screening process. She had a previous history of placental insufficiency which was diagnosed at 38 weeks gestation following doppler wave form. Induction of labour was attempted using prostin pessaries. Fetal distress was observed on the cardiotocograph tracing, and an emergency lower segment caesarean section was performed. The live male infant weighed 2.350kg (5lb 4oz), Staphylococcus aureus septicaemia was suspected. He is alive and well.

Present pregnancy

The mother booked at ten weeks gestation. The plan of care was to perform serial scans from 28 weeks gestation, maintain a fetal movement chart, perform serial doppler ultrasound techniques and cardiotocograph traces.

The volume of liquor was judged to be reduced at 36 weeks gestation and at 38 weeks gestation. Amniotic fluid volume is indicative of fetal and/or placental function. Druzin (1992) proposed that a single amniotic fluid pocket of 1cm or less was highly suggestive of intrauterine growth retardation. An amniotic fluid index has also been developed which assesses the likelihood of perinatal morbidity in spite of a non-stress test and absence of fetal heart decelerations (Phelan et al, 1987). When the tracing below was recorded the mother had reported reduced fetal movements. Asymmetrical intrauterine growth retardation was reported on scan.

Discussion of the trace (Fig. 6.2)

This is a good quality trace. The 25 minute trace shown has been extracted from a trace lasting 40 minutes. It illustrates a baseline fetal heart rate of between 130 and 135 bpm. Therefore, as the baseline fetal heart rate variation is only 5 bpm this indicates stretches of decreased long-term variability. This is normally associated with sleep

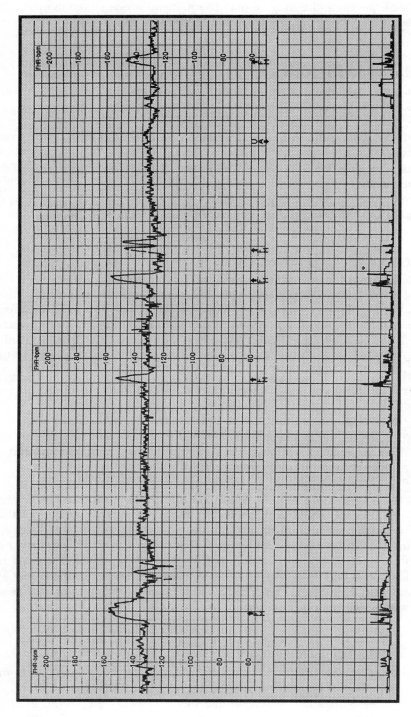

Fig. 6.2: Case study one

pattern. Nevertheless, there are accelerations with fetal movements and four fetal movements have been recorded within a 20-minute period. There is little uterine activity documented. The features which are reassuring are the accelerations and the fetal movements. However, in order to assess the significance of the decreased long-term variability, further traces need to be scrutinized. It would have been inappropriate to have come to any conclusions about this fetus' well-being on this trace alone.

Outcome

Further traces demonstrated normal variability. This woman was very anxious as a result of her previous labour experience so an elective caesarean section was planned at term at her request. Meanwhile, spontaneous onset of labour occurred at 39+ weeks gestation. Although an epidural was sited the mother experienced a very painful latent stage and continued to be very anxious throughout and thus requested an emergency caesarean section. A live male was delivered weighing 2.990kg (6lb 9oz).

Case study two

This woman was a 35 year old gravida 2 para 1 who smoked two cigarettes per day. She had suffered a previous unexplained intrauterine death at 41+ weeks gestation. Post-mortem was refused by the parents so the cause of death could not be fully investigated. However, because of her history an intensified programme of antenatal screening was implemented.

Present pregnancy

All antenatal care was to be performed in the hospital setting including serial scans, doppler studies and maintenance of a fetal movement chart from 28 weeks gestation. The mother was very frightened throughout the pregnancy and constant support and reassurance was readily available.

Discussion of the trace (Fig. 6.3)

This trace was recorded at 36 weeks gestation and is of good quality. This is a 28 minute extract from a trace of 45 minutes. A baseline fetal heart rate of 125-140 bpm is shown. This baseline range demonstrates good variability. Five accelerations can be observed associated with fetal movements. Little uterine activity is recorded. This is a reassuring trace which indicates that the fetus appears to be adequately oxygenated at this time, but to ensure continued well-being serial cardiotocograph traces were performed.

Outcome

It was decided that because of this woman's previous stillbirth induction of labour would be carried out prior to term. At 38 weeks gestation her membranes were artificially ruptured. A live baby girl was delivered weighing 3.250kg (7lb 3oz).

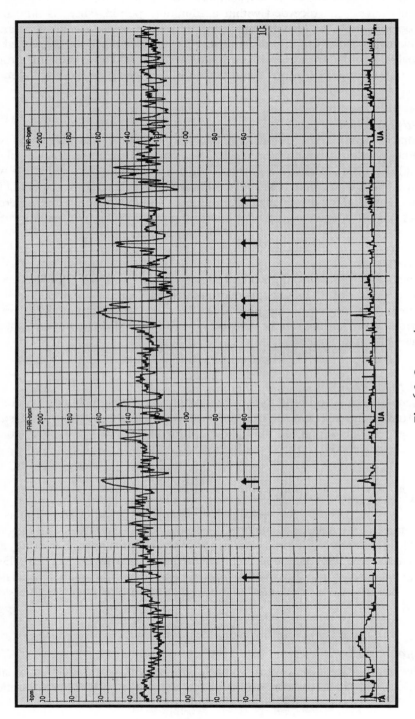

Fig. 6.3: Case study two

Case study three

This woman is 20 years old and a primigravida. At 15 weeks gestation she was diagnosed by ultrasound scan as having a twin pregnancy. She developed a raised blood pressure and urinary tract infection at 31 weeks gestation. Intrauterine growth retardation was suspected clinically and confirmed by ultrasound at 33 weeks gestation.

Discussion of trace (Fig. 6.4)

This a good quality trace and is an extract of 19 minutes from a 40 minute trace. It demonstrates simultaneous recording of both fetal heart rates. Both fetuses have normal baseline fetal heart rates and variability.

Twin 1 (US 1) has baseline fetal heart rate rising to between 160 and 165 bpm after the first five minutes. Good variability is observed. Altogether six accelerations are recorded corresponding with uterine activity and fetal movements.

Twin II (US 2) has a lower baseline fetal heart rate of between 130 and 140 bpm. Good variability is observed. In total seven accelerations are recorded, four of which are in conjunction with twin 1.

Some uterine activity is recorded following calibration of the uterine transducer. This is a reassuring trace which indicates that at this time both fetuses are well oxygenated. Observation of these fetuses continued for the remainder of this pregnancy on a weekly basis.

Outcome

Induction of labour was performed at 37 weeks gestation due to a rise in blood pressure which was raised further in labour.

Twin Is heart rate was recorded by fetal scalp electrode and was delivered by Kiellands forceps delivery, weighing 2.270kg (5lb). Twin IIs heart rate was recorded by external ultrasound transducer, delivered by Neville Barnes forceps weighing 2.400kg (5lb 5oz). The labour lasted a total of 5 hours 50 mins total.

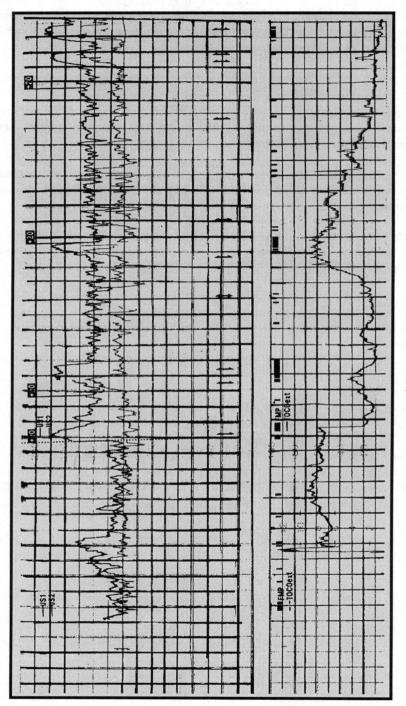

Fig. 6.4: Case study three

Case study four

A 28-year-old primigravida who booked at 12+ weeks gestation with no relevant history.

Present pregnancy

At booking a singleton pregnancy was diagnosed. An ultrasound scan confirmed her menstrual history. The protocol for her Consultant was to commence a fetal movement chart at 26 weeks gestation. At this time the pregnancy was progressing well and all observations were normal. She was admitted at 29 weeks gestation to the delivery suite with a history of decreased fetal movements for three days and a history of losing clear fluid per vaginam for one week. A speculum examination was performed but there was no evidence of rupture of membranes. A cardiotocograph was performed, a section of which is illustrated below.

Discussion of trace (Fig. 6.5)

This trace is of good quality. A total of 45 minutes of tracing was recorded although only 12 minutes is reproduced. The baseline range is of good variability. The baseline rate is 150–160 bpm.

There are several rises of ten bpm or more above the baseline which last for ten seconds or more. This is normal for the preterm fetus of 30 weeks gestation. (A rise of 15 bpm for 15 seconds is normal for a fetus of more than 30 weeks gestation.) Also of note, there are several decreases in the baseline rate but these are transitory and do not last more than ten seconds – this too, is common in normal fetuses of 20–30 weeks gestation (Pillai and James, 1990). Therefore what on first glance could have been described as a disconcerting deceleration is normal in fetuses of between 20 and 30 weeks gestation. Some weak uterine activity can be observed.

Outcome

This woman was reassured and discharged home after this to be reviewed in the antenatal clinic one week later. Sadly, she was readmitted six days later by the community midwife with a further history of reduced fetal movements. The fetal heart had not been heard by the community midwife. Ultrasound scan confirmed intrauterine fetal death. Labour was induced and a stillborn female baby was delivered which weighed 1.310 kg (2lb 15oz). No external abnormalities were apparent, although the placenta showed evidence of infarction. The post-mortem report found no significant internal or external anatomical abnormalities. Intrauterine death was assessed as being of 12–48 hours duration.

Comment

This case history demonstrates the complexity of antenatal incidents as this intrauterine death followed a normal cardiotocograph trace only six days previously. The mother's concern was justified and should remind professionals of the importance of listening

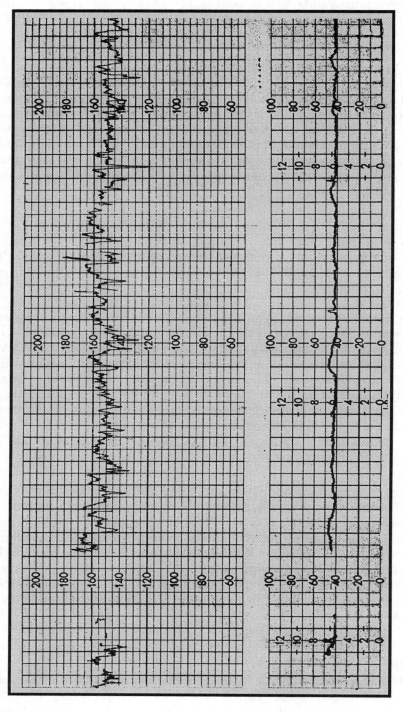

Fig. 6.5: Case study four

carefully to the mother. Despite the use of cardiotocography, in this instance the mother was a better judge of fetal well-being.

Case study five

This 34 year old lady is a gravida 6 para 3+2 and originates from Central Africa. During 1989 she experienced two miscarriages both at 12 weeks gestation. She had raised blood pressure during her next pregnancy in 1988 but delivered normally in the UK at 36 weeks gestation. She delivered a live baby boy who weighed 2.025kg (4 lb 10 oz) who made normal progress.

Her next pregnancy in 1990, although well antenatally, culminated in an emergency caesarean section for shoulder presentation. She delivered a live boy who weighed 3.00kg (6 lb 13oz) who is alive and well.

Her last pregnancy was in 1992 when she again had raised blood pressure antenatally. She had a normal delivery in Central Africa and had a live boy who weighed 2.47 kg (5 lb 7 oz) who is alive and well.

Present pregnancy

This woman returned to England from Central Africa when she was 36+ weeks gestation and booked soon afterwards. At this time she reported reduced fetal movements. Intrauterine growth retardation was clinically suspected. Antenatal cardiotocograph tracings were performed. Ultrasound scan indicated a very mature placenta and doppler studies demonstrated high resistance flow. Close observation continued with the woman attending as a day case in the Antenatal Assessment area, twice a week.

At 39 weeks gestation cardiotocograph tracing recorded a fetal tachycardia of 180 bpm rising to 220 bpm accompanied by reduced variability. The maternal temperature spiked to 38.6°C. The midwife in the Antenatal Assessment area queried malaria particularly as the mother had never taken anti-malarial drugs, and because of her history and the clinical presentation. The maternal temperature continued to rise. Malaria was confirmed from blood samples.

Discussion of trace (Fig. 6.6)

This is a good quality tracing using ultrasound to record the fetal heart rate. The presented portion of a 60 minute trace is of 29 minute duration. The baseline rate is 175–180 bpm. However, in the latter part of the illustrated section there is a period where the fetal heart rate rises above the 200 bpm which is the limit of the machine's recording capability. This machine did not have the facility to record fetal movements. The variability is reduced. There are no significant accelerations and no decelerations are recorded. Some uterine activity can be observed.

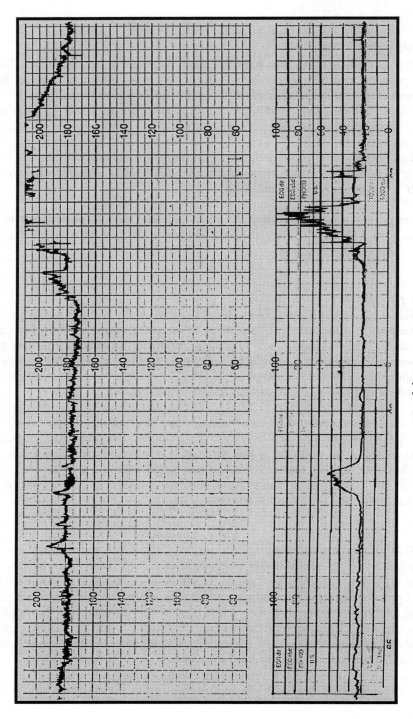

Fig. 6.6: Case study Five

Outcome

An emergency lower segment caesarean section was performed immediately following this tracing. A live girl of 39 weeks gestation was delivered, with Apgar scores of 9 at one minute and 10 at five minutes, weighing 2240kg (4lb 15oz). The mother made a good recovery with anti-malarial treatment. No problems were anticipated with the baby.

KEY POINTS

•   The search for an antenatal test which can predict fetal morbidity and mortality continues.

•   The non-stress test has largely taken over from the contraction stress test, however, the biophysical profile provides much more data about the acute and chronic state of the fetus.

•   All antenatal tests need to be viewed as part of the total care of the woman.

•   The midwife has a key role in care of the woman with an 'at risk' pregnancy. Her involvement is not only in the carrying out of investigations but in the holistic care of the woman and her partner.

CHAPTER SEVEN

The Electronic Fetal Heart Rate Monitoring Debate

This chapter presents some of the arguments surrounding electronic fetal heart rate monitoring. It is the dialogue of a conversation actually had by the authors. It is written in narrative (rather than essay style) to add interest to the debate and the book. It is also intended to present the discussion in a way that practitioners might utilize and develop to stimulate further debate in clinical practice.

JB   'The trouble with the debate about the use of electronic fetal monitoring is that it has been mainly concerned with the prevention of cerebral palsy, birth asphyxia and the reduction of perinatal mortality and morbidity[1,2,3,4] . This work is very important, of course, but there are other issues which have to be addressed as well.'

JW   'What sort of things are you thinking about?'

JB   'Well, with any intervention, one of the first things midwives and doctors must consider is consent, and I mean informed maternal consent. Do midwives inform women of the disadvantages as well as the advantages? Like the higher risk of operative delivery[5], that their position will be restricted and that it would therefore be difficult to have a delivery in an alternative position[6]; that the evidence for the relationship between abnormal traces and birth asphyxia is very tenuous and also that it does not significantly reduce perinatal mortality or morbidity.[7,8,9] Midwives must inform mothers of these facts according to the UKCC "Code of Professional Conduct" and "Exercising Accountability".[10,11] '

JW   'The trouble is that I think women have caught on to this idea that if they are put on to a monitor their baby is safe. They will put up with being uncomfortable or in a restricted position because they have real trust in the monitor, believing it will pick up anything wrong with their baby early enough to do something about it.[12] '

JB   'It also gives them a sense of security that when the midwife leaves the delivery room there is still surveillance of their baby. Midwives must be careful that the monitor is not used to be a substitute for midwifery care.[13,14] The idea can creep in that a woman will be all right during a coffee break because she is attached to a monitor.'

JW   'I think you're right because it could be only too easy when units are short staffed to use monitors in an inappropriate way. Midwives must be aware of the dangers of using monitoring as a caregiver substitute.[6] The CTG machine cannot make any decisions for the midwife, it is only as good as the midwife who is responsible for it. Not only that, but there is the problem that CTG machines have the potential to de-skill midwives, not merely in their ability to record the fetal heart in labour by auscultation, but also because of the unique position of the midwife being sensitive and aware of the total picture and care of the women. If a midwife is "with woman" then she is observing the more subtle changes over a period of time and she is therefore not just looking at one aspect. Being aware of the whole picture means that she can assess whether the woman is in a poor position or is progressing normally.'

JB   'It is more difficult to provide such care when the CTG gives the midwife "permission" to leave the room in order to care for other labouring women. The machine begins to take on the role of mechanical observer but it is so limited in what it can observe.'

JW   'There are legal and ethical considerations to take into account and it is unacceptable to use monitors in this way. If a midwife puts a woman on a monitor she is accepting responsibility. For the monitor to be of any use, someone must be available at all times to interpret the trace and initiate the most appropriate management. The midwife is still accountable if she leaves the room with the woman on the monitor unsupervised and an abnormal fetal heart rate pattern occurs which really requires immediate action.'

JB   'So should midwives be using electronic monitors if they are not able to be present to interpret the traces? Is it therefore acceptable for a woman on a monitor to be left? If the trace is reassuring and the woman is low-risk, electronic monitoring is unnecessary. If fetal monitoring is used it should be on women who are high-risk and they should not be left. The legal implication is that if the woman on a CTG is left for any reason this should be recorded and documented on the trace so that every minute can be accounted for.'

JW   'There are not only problems with interpretation of the CTG but also with what actually causes cerebral palsy. When does the insult which results in cerebral palsy occur? Chronic hypoxia, or an acute hypoxic insult, during pregnancy can result in similar damage to that which occurs with a severe acute hypoxic insult during labour. It could even be a combination of problems of oxygenation both antenatally and in labour.[1,15,16] '

JB   The trouble is that if permanent hypoxic damage has occurred in pregnancy but is not fatal, the added stress of labour may in such compromised fetuses result in fetal distress. The hypoxic damage is then attributed to intrapartum events when really the damage occurred long before.[1,15,16] '

JW   'If monitoring is used in labour and the damage has already occurred antenatally, then there is nothing anyone can do and monitoring is merely a case of shutting the stable door after the horse has bolted.'

JB   'It is interesting to note that the Grant research[9], which isn't new, identifies that most of the permanent damage due to hypoxia has occurred not in labour but long before sometime during the antenatal period.'

JW   'There is actually evidence to suggest that only eight per cent of cerebral palsy is associated with asphyxia during labour and at delivery. Midwives should not forget that such an association of cause and effect cannot always be made.[17] In other words, the eight per cent of cerebral palsy which is associated with asphyxia during labour and at delivery is not necessarily caused as a direct result of intrapartum events alone.'

JB   'The figure of eight per cent is so low it is now thought that fetal heart rate monitoring couldn't reduce the rates of cerebral palsy.[18]'

JW   'It would be helpful if the length of time from the commencement of an abnormal CTG to permanent damage could be determined. However, some fetuses deteriorate faster than others. Fleischer[19] did attempt to identify the length of time from late and variable decelerations and loss of baseline variability to acidosis but acidosis has not been found to be a good indicator of long-term neurological outcome.[20,21]'

JB   'Looking at it from a reassuring point of view, it has been suggested that a normal reactive trace indicates a fetal reserve of seven days.[22,23]'

JW   'Electronic monitoring was thought to be a sufficiently reliable test. In labour it would identify those babies at risk of hypoxic ischaemic encephalopathy. It was believed that action could then be taken to prevent long-term damage. It was considered that in preventing hypoxic ischaemic encephalopathy, long-term damage such as cerebral palsy could also be prevented. However, not all cases of hypoxic ischaemic encephalopathy result in cerebral palsy and not all cerebral palsy is a result of hypoxic ischaemic encephalopathy.[1,18] CTG monitoring is fraught with problems due to the complexity of traces and their interpretation.[5,8,24,25,26]'

JB   'It seems strange that despite all the evidence that has accumulated over the years and the review of its use in *Effective Care in Pregnancy and Childbirth*[27] which suggests that electronic fetal monitoring has not reduced cerebral palsy nor the perinatal mortality rate, it is still routinely used. It probably continues to be widely used because there is a belief that the use of high-technology must be better than human expertise.'

JW   'It might also be because it sounds so plausible and because it provides carers with control. Using cardiotocograph machines means women have attached to the monitor. It therefore provides a degree of power and along with other interventions such as epidurals[28] restricts the woman's choices and mobility. Using the monitor demonstrates the need for expert knowledge and that the professionals know what is best.'

JB   'One of the reasons electronic fetal heart rate monitoring has not been rationalized in its use is that it has a controlling effect for both the obstetricians over the midwives and women and the midwives themselves over the women. The use of the monitor limits the type and options of care that can be given and may be why telemetry has never been widely used.'

JW   'I am deeply concerned about the controlling effect of EFM. I'm sure there must be a place for such monitoring. A normal trace is a reliable reassurance that the fetal outcome will be good.[29] Many units now use an admission test where the fetal heart is recorded for about 30–40 minutes. Rest cycles may mean the trace needs to be continued or repeated to ensure that the trace is reactive and not abnormal.[30]'

JB   'The admission test is used not only to identify that the fetus is normal and therefore the outcome of labour is likely to be normal but also as baseline to determine deviations from normal.'

JW   'In this respect the work on recording of blood pressure may have lessons to teach us. It is unlikely even in well people that the blood pressure would remain constant throughout a 24-hour period and that it might be more useful to take mean recordings than the odd one off recording. Similarly, the admission test in labour is only a small picture of the fetal heart rate. It is used as a contraction stress test. It might be that the point of admission is the worst time to record the fetal heart rate trace because we all know of the effect that the stress of admission has on women. It is common for women to come into hospital with a history of regular painful contractions and then, following admission, the contractions wear off. After a time, once the woman has settled on labour ward, the contractions recommence.[31,32]

JB   'It would then seem more appropriate if the fetal heart was recorded electronically for a fixed period some two hours after admission and hopefully by then some women, of course, would have delivered!'

JW   'The other problem with the admission test is that midwives are working from a medical background where a baseline to identify change is deemed necessary. Labour is a dynamic event where circumstances continually change. It may not be possible to clearly identify a baseline during labour. But it might be useful to know the baseline fetal heart rate antenatally in order to make a comparison. It should, however, be remembered that gestation and other factors affect fetal heart rates as do fetal movements which also change during labour.[33]'

JB   'If the fetal heart rate is monitored on admission it is really being used as a contraction stress test. This is of doubtful use as well because the strength of contractions progressively increases throughout labour. Can it be assumed that if a fetus can cope with contractions early in labour, it will automatically cope with contractions that are stronger later in labour.'

JW   'Whether the admission test is useful or valid in determining a baseline fetal heart rate the real difficulty occurs when there is an abnormal trace. The specificity [the ability to test for fetuses who are not distressed] is good but the sensitivity [the ability to test for fetuses who are distressed] is poor. So the test provides a large number of false positives. When using EFM in conjunction with FBS it has been found that 61 per cent of distressed fetuses could be detected but 95 per cent of those identified as distressed during labour were not found to be asphyxiated at delivery.[34]'

JB   'That's right, and that's why there is an increase in operative deliveries without benefit to the baby when fetal heart rate monitoring is used.[5,7]'

JW   'So in whose interest is electronic fetal monitoring being performed? Is it for the mother and her partner, for the reassurance they enjoy when hearing and "seeing" their baby's heart beating? Or is it for the midwife, to have a machine to record the fetal heart, and supposedly release her for other responsibilities? Or is it for the obstetrician and other carers, including the midwife, as a form of protection against litigation?'

JB   'Both midwives and doctors seem to consider that monitoring the fetal heart rate gives them some sort of legal protection.[35,36,37] Monitoring at least provides some evidence or statement of the care that has been given and confirmation that the fetal heart rate was really recorded.'

JW   'Yes, because the trace is so visual, continuous and recorded by a machine. The danger is that it is perceived to be a more accurate representation of what has happened in labour rather than the midwife's manually recorded and documented observations.'

JB   'It's strange really because for legal reasons the trace may not actually offer any security against litigation at all. Quite the reverse, in fact, because a poor trace is worse than not having a trace at all.[35,37] For the trace to be used as evidence to support the midwife's provision of care it must be an accurate recording. There must be a written record of any action (or no action) taken following interpretations of the trace.[35,37] The responsibility for the good working order of the monitoring machinery is essentially that of the midwife. The trace must also have documented on it the correct time and every single event that takes place, however inconsequential it may seem. Each minute of the trace should be accounted for by the midwife so that it may be accurately interpreted and appropriate action taken. Who would you, then, say is responsible for the interpretation of an abnormal trace?'

JW   'The "Midwives Rules"[38], "Code of Professional Conduct"[39] and "The Scope of Professional Practice"[40] all make it clear that if a midwife accepts the care of a woman on a cardiotocographic monitor that she must be competent in its full use and therefore the midwife must be capable of interpreting the trace. It is the midwife's responsibility that the woman receives the care she wants and the care which the midwife believes to be in the best interests of the mother and her fetus. It should, however, be recognized that midwives are the experts in normality and have a duty to refer the abnormal, but this is no excuse for lack of skills. Midwives are responsible for their actions at all times.[39] '

JB   'There are, of course, difficulties in interpretation of traces. Professionals cannot agree on the interpretation of traces. Obstetricians have been given the same cardiotocographic traces to interpret and have demonstrated a wide variation of opinion. The same obstetricians, shown the same traces at a later date, made different interpretations to their original statement.[41] '

JW   'This, of course, throws doubt on the reliability of the interpretation of the trace. If obstetricians demonstrate both inter-observer and intra-observer differences in interpreting the same trace, how does a midwife identify what is in the best interests of the women in her care?'

JB   'The midwife may feel she is competent at caring for a mother on a cardiotocographic machine but she may not be fully up-to-date on electronic fetal heart rate monitoring.[14] '

JW   'Research is continually finding out new information which may or may not be compatible with current practice. However, there is always a delay in implementing research-based findings into practice as the research on electronic monitoring demonstrates. What the midwife will be judged on in law of course is the Bolam Test. Where the standards recognized as acceptable are those "of the ordinary skilled man exercising and professing to have that skill."[42] Man in this context meaning midwife.'

JB   'But if the research on traces is inconclusive and the medical profession cannot determine which traces require action and which do not, should the midwife be accepting responsibility for women on cardiotocograph machines?'

JW   'I think the midwife has got to know her real legal responsibilities in accepting care for a woman on a cardiotocographic machine. Certainly in respect of record-keeping, ensuring the quality of the trace, and in ensuring the technology is being used in the best interests of the mother and fetus.[10,11,38,40,43,44,45]   In addition, she has responsibility for the good working order of the machinery and to take appropriate action if there is any doubt.[35] It is also the midwife's responsibility to ensure that traces are seen by the appropriate person in the event of the midwife herself not being certain on the interpretation of a trace.[11]

JB   'It is then true to say that a midwife must be able to identify a normal trace, and that she must refer any traces which are not normal to someone who can interpret them and can act upon their interpretation, to the satisfaction of the midwife. It should also be remembered that the midwife has a duty to document all such events in the mothers notes.[38,45] '

JW 'There is, of course, the question of whether electronic fetal heart rate monitoring is appropriate for all women. What has happened in practice fits in with the notion that once one intervention is used there is a cascade of intervention.[46] The very act of strapping a woman to a monitor means that the woman is subjected to a very different type of care from that which she would receive if the fetal heart was recorded intermittently. The restrictions imposed on the woman by continuous monitoring make it more difficult for them to divert her attention by frequently changing position, increasing her need for analgesia and so affecting the respirator function of the baby. Delivery in an alternative position is difficult and there is the evidence of the increased forceps and caesarean section rates.'

JB 'It might be more useful if CTGs were not interpreted in isolation but considered alongside fetal blood samples and the complete clinical picture.[47,48] '

JW 'It is worrying that some units are still using CTG without fetal blood sampling.[49] Decisions of management should not be made solely on the information obtained from a CTG because it is so unreliable.'

JB 'It is likely then that electronic heart rate monitoring has been directed into the wrong area of care. Perhaps it does have a place but it should be more focused on antenatal care as well as women who are high-risk during labour.'

JW 'You mean that energy should be concentrated on identifying those babies at risk of permanent hypoxic damage antenatally and then decide what the appropriate management should be, before the hypoxia causes long-term problems?'

JB 'But then hypoxic injury can occur at any gestation and therefore it becomes a question of when is it appropriate to commence screening high-risk fetuses with electronic fetal heart rate monitoring? At what gestation is it ethical to monitor the fetal heart rate and make the decision on the interpretation of the trace to intervene and deliver the baby acknowledging that the normal preterm fetal heart rate trace is different from that of a normal term fetus.'

JW 'There is certainly a potential for great ethical and clinical dilemmas. For instance a 24 week fetus could be identified on CTG as demonstrating signs of serious hypoxic compromise. Should it be delivered with all the problems of caring for the extremely preterm infant or should it be allowed to die naturally in utero?'

JB 'The parents might appreciate the opportunity to hold their baby alive, even though it may die or be left permanently damaged, rather than leave it to die in utero. It could be that despite fetal monitoring the outcome for the fetus would be the same but parents might have the choice of waiting for their baby to die in utero or holding it in their arms until it dies. It seems that this is another area of personal morality where there is no one right answer.'

JW 'It could make it very difficult for parents to participate in deciding when it is appropriate to intervene and instigate care that may or may not be successful, when their expectations of medical intervention are so high. One must also consider the long-term effect of any such intervention may have on that woman's reproductive health. A caesarean performed for a 24-week fetus who does not survive, and before the lower segment has properly formed, has more serious implications for future pregnancies than a caesarean at term.[50] This brings us back to the importance of gaining informed consent.'

JB 'There is even some evidence that antenatal electronic monitoring of the fetal heart rate has not been successful in decreasing morbidity and mortality. A study was performed where some antenatal CTGs were hidden and some were reviewed. Action was taken for patients on whom the traces were reviewed if the trace was considered suspicious of hypoxia. There was in fact a higher mortality rate for those babies whose CTGs were acted upon rather than those whose CTGs were hidden.[51]'

JW 'In that case it could be that the very act of using antenatal CTGs might mean that babies are delivered earlier than they would have been if there had been no antenatal CTGs performed and that as a result they could be doing more harm than good by increasing perinatal morbidity. This could also possibly be true for recording the fetal heart by ultrasound rather than directly with the use of the scalp electrode. In all our research for this book we have found nothing that addresses the issue of safety and the use of ultrasound in labour to record the fetal heart. Recently the World Health Organization[52] recommended that ultrasound should not be used routinely because its safety is in doubt. It may be that CTG, ultrasound and scanning machines are not comparable but ultrasound monitoring can be used during labour for great lengths of time. Does it have an accumulative effect? Is it like cooking at 100°C for four hours rather than one hour at 180°C?'

JB 'Do you think it would be possible for midwives to refuse to electronically monitor the fetal heart of low-risk women in hospitals where there are policies which dictate the recording of an admission test at least?'

JW 'If midwives are providing individualized care there should not be rigid policies but guidelines which give direction. Parameters of care for women which allow flexibility should be identified by obstetricians and midwives. Care should be given in the best interests of women and sensitive to the individual needs. Information should be given to assist in choice and consent obtained for any care women receive.[53]'

JB 'Midwives are fighting for the right not to perform an amniotomy routinely. Perhaps the time has come for them to push for a reduction in the use of fetal heart rate monitoring, too.'

JW 'Certainly as intermittent auscultation of the fetal heart is as reliable as the CTG[54], then midwives should be putting forward a strong case to decrease the routine use of monitors.'

JB   'The trouble is that midwives have to walk that very difficult line between hospital policy and the best interests of the client.[11,39] The midwife has to ask herself to whom is she primarily responsible. Theoretically, first and foremost, she is accountable to the woman but practically, it is exceptionally hard for the midwife to be the woman's advocate if she is at risk of losing her job.'

JB   'We've now come full circle with this debate. It brings us back yet again to the difficulties of ensuring informed consent.'

JW   'Informed consent becomes a huge ethical dilemma, when electronic fetal heart rate monitoring is used. The whole issue of monitoring is problematic and yet it is still "perceived" to be a reliable safeguard for the baby. Action is taken on the information provided, however as we have debated, the evidence of any benefit is inconclusive and maternal and fetal morbidity is no less.'

JB   'To date there has been a lot of financial commitment to electronic fetal heart rate monitoring. Money has already been spent on the machinery and continues to be invested in technologic advances. Therefore it still needs to be questioned whose interests EFM serves?'

KEY FACTS

- Midwives must obtain informed consent from the mother before the electronic fetal heart rate monitor is used.

- When electronic fetal heart rate monitoring is used the midwife is accountable for the care a woman receives.

- Midwives must ensure that care is always given in the best interests of mothers and babies.

- Midwives must be fully trained in the use of cardiotocographs and interpretation of traces.

- Midwives must ensure that electronic monitoring does not result in the loss of skills or sub-standard levels of care.

- Midwives must ensure that all events and decisions are recorded on the CTG trace and in mothers notes.

- EFM does not significantly reduce perinatal mortality or morbidity but increases the caesarean section rate.

- Intermittent auscultation is equally as good as EFM at predicting fetal wellbeing.

- The relationship between a pathological trace and an asphyxiated baby is tenuous.

References

1. Hull and Dodd, 1991
2. Prentice and Lind, 1987
3. Freeman, 1990
4. Anthony and Levene, 1990
5. Grant, 1989
6. Garcia et al, 1985
7. MacDonald et al, 1985
8. Ellison et al 1991
9. Grant et al, 1989
10. UKCC, 1992a
11. UKCC, 1989
12. Starkman 1976
13. Tucker 1992
14. Cooke 1992
15. Williams et al, 1993
16. Boylan, 1987
17. Bryce, Stanley and Blair, 1989
18. Carter, Haverkamp and Merenstein, 1993
19. Fleischer et al, 1982
20. Dennis et al, 1989
21. Ruth and Raivio, 1988
22. Evertson et al, 1979
23. Gibbons and Nagle, 1980
24. Rosen and Dickinson, 1993
25. Spencer, 1993
26. Curzen et al, 1984
27. Chalmers et al, 1989
28. Wagner 1986
29. Druzin, 1992
30. Gibb and Arulkumaran, 1992
31. Crowther et al, 1989
32. Naattgeboren, 1989
33. Spencer and Johnson, 1986
34. Van den Berg et al, 1987
35. Symonds, 1993
36. Ennis, Clark and Grudzinskas 1991
37. Capstick and Edwards, 1991
38. UKCC, 1993b
39. UKCC, 1992a
40. UKCC, 1992b
41. Barrett et al, 1990
42. Dimond, 1990
43. UKCC, 1994
44. UKCC, 1994
45. UKCC, 1993a
46. World Health Organisation, 1985
47. Spencer, 1992
48. Devoe, 1988
49. Wheble et al, 1989
50. Keirse, 1989
51. Grant and Mohide, 1982
52. Tsechkowski, 1993
53. Department of Health, 1993
54. Paine et al, 1992

All the references shown above can be found in full in the reference list at the end of this book.

CHAPTER EIGHT

Epilogue

The prospective trials of EFM have not demonstrated the benefits which had been hoped for (Shy, Larson and Luthy, 1987; Grant, 1989; Thacker, 1991). The reasons for this have been postulated to be:

1. Intrapartum perinatal asphyxia as a cause for cerebral palsy occurs only in 1 to 2 per 10,000 term labours. The technology cannot affect such small numbers.

2. Electronic fetal monitoring is a poor predictor of fetal asphyxia.

3. Catastrophic events such a severe abruption that can cause asphyxial damage happen so rapidly that deliveries cannot be effected before damage occurs (Carter, Haverkamp and Merenstein, 1993).

4. Hypoxic injury can occur antenatally before labour commences.

5. Hypoxic injury may occur because of an existing neurological abnormality (Freeman, 1990).

Glossary

artefact   irregularities on a tracing shown as dots or lines due
                                       to electrical interference or poor fetal heart rate
                                       signal

acceleration   transitory increase of at least 15 bpm above the
                                       baseline rate and lasting 15 seconds or more.

baseline variability   variation of the baseline fetal heart rate.

biophysical profile   assessment of fetal condition using a variety of
                                       observations namely, fetal heart rate patterns, fetal
                                       breathing movements, reflex activity, amniotic fluid
                                       volume and placental grading. Each feature can be
                                       given a score which collectively assesses degree of
                                       risk to the fetus.

bradycardia   baseline bradycardia is defined as a fetal heart rate of
                                       110 bpm or below. It is pathological if it is below 100
                                       bpm.

cardiotocography (CTG)   graphical representation of the fetal heart rate and
                                       uterine contractions

contraction stress test (CST)   observation of fetal heart rate patterns using electronic
                                       fetal heart monitoring in response to induced uterine
                                       contractions, i.e. using oxytocin, nipple stimulation.

deceleration   temporary decrease of 15 bpm or more below the
                                       baseline rate and lasting 15 seconds or more.

doppler ultrasound   type of ultrasound used in electronic fetal heart rate
                                       monitors, can also be used to assess blood flow in
                                       fetal and placental vessels.

early deceleration   deceleration which occurs in conjunction with a
                                       uterine contraction.

EFM   electronic fetal monitoring.

late deceleration   deceleration which occurs after the onset of a
                                       contraction.

long-term variability	rhythmical variation of 15–20 bpm seen in the baseline rate over one minute.
nonstress test (NST)	observation of the fetal heart and acceleration in response to fetal movements or Braxton Hicks contractions using electronic fetal heart rate monitoring.
overshooting	accelerations which occur immediately after a deceleration.
saltatory	increased variability in the fetal heart rate, variability rate of more than 25 bpm.
short-term variability	normal variation of between five and ten bpm between each heart beat.
shouldering	accelerations which occur immediately before a deceleration.
tachycardia	baseline tachycardia is defined as a fetal heart rate of 150 bpm or more in a fetus at term. It is said to be moderate if it is between 150 and 170 bpm and severe if it is greater than 170 bpm.
telemetry	radio waves which can be used to record uterine contractions and the fetal heart rate by remote control. Rates are transmitted to a receiver and printed on to graph paper after the monitor has processed information.
tocotransducer	instrument which monitors frequency and duration of contractions by means of a pressure-sensing device applied to the abdomen.
ultrasound	high frequency sound waves form beams which are partly reflected at each boundary between tissues, e.g. closure of fetal heart valves. Using an ultrasound transducer (which transforms vibrations from electrical charges into ultrasound waves) the fetal heart can be monitored.
variable decelerations	decelerations that are not consistently late or early. They do not have a regular pattern and vary in onset.

Electronic Monitoring Checklist

Prior to commencement of a fetal heart tracing the following points should be observed.

The fetal monitor
- Is the graph paper inserted correctly?
- Is there sufficient paper?
- Are the transducers inserted into the correct sockets?

The tocotransducer
- Is the transducer firmly held in place in the fundal region of the uterus?
- Has the transducer been applied to the abdomen without gel?
- Has the pen been calibrated between contractions?

The ultrasound transducer
- Has aqueous gel been smeared to its underside?
- Has the fetal heart rate been heard and recorded on the graph paper?
- Is the belt holding the transducer in place?
- If the fetal monitor has an oscilloscope, does a consistent wave form appear?

The fetal scalp electrode (if applied)
- Are the wires of the scalp electrode connected to the leg plate?
- Has the underside of the leg plate been smeared with aqueous gel?
- Is the leg plate securely applied to the woman's thigh?
- Is the fetal scalp electrode attached to the presenting part of the fetus?

Record-keeping
Has the following been written on the graph paper?

- The woman's name
- Hospital number
- Date
- The time when monitoring commenced

- Ultrasound transducer or fetal scalp electrode?
- Any significant details for example, state of membranes, high-risk conditions, e.g. pregnancy-induced hypertension, diabetes, cervical dilatation and station of presenting part.

The following incidents need also to be recorded on the graph paper when appropriate:

- position of mother and when position is changed
- when vaginal examinations are performed
- medication given
- observations – temperature, pulse, respirations, blood pressure
- use of bedpan
- oxygen administered
- fetal movements
- pushing during the second stage of labour
- change in mode of monitoring for example, application of a fetal scalp electrode
- adjustments made to equipment for example, repositioning of transducers.

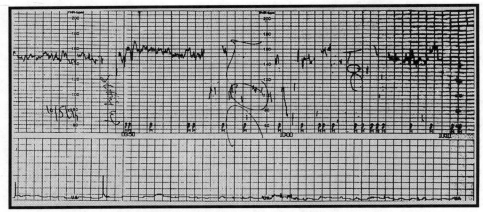

Fig. A1: Trace illustrating record keeping

LOC   Loss of contact
FM   Fetal movement

(Some monitors have a data input device which can be used to record pertinent information on the graph paper for example, date, time, fetal movements.)

References

Anthony, M.Y., Levene, M.I. (1990). 'An assessment of the benefits of intrapartum fetal monitoring'. *Developmental Medicine and Child Neurology*, 32, 6, June, pp.547–53.

Barrett, J.F.R., Jarvis, G.J., MacDonald, H.N., Buchan, P.C., Tyrell, S.N., Lilford, R.J. (1990). 'Inconsistencies in clinical decisions in obstetrics'. *Lancet*, 336, 8714, pp. 549–51.

Beard, R.W., Filshie, G.M., Knight, C.A., Roberts, G.M. (1971). 'The significance of the changes in the continuous fetal heart rate in the first stage of labour'. *Journal of Obstetrics and Gynaecololgy of the British Commonwealth*. 78, pp.865–81.

Boylan, P. (1987). 'Intrapartum fetal monitoring'. *Fetal Monitoring – Clinical Obstetrics and Gynaecology – International Practice and Research*, 1, March, pp. 73–95.

Boylan, P. (1991). 'Liquor assessment: meconium and oligohydamnios'. In: Spencer, J.A.D. (Ed). *Fetal Monitoring*. Oxford: Oxford University Press.

British Medical Journal 289, 6455, Nov 17, 345-1347.

Bryce, R., Stanley, F., Blair, E. (1989). 'The effects of intrapartum care on the risk of impairments in childhood'. In: Chalmers, I., Enkin, M., Keirse, M.J.N.C. (Eds). *Effective Care in Pregnancy and Childbirth*. Oxford: Oxford University Press.

Caldeyro-Barcia, R., Mendez-Bauer, C., Poseior, J.J. et al (1966) 'Control of human fetal heart rate during labor'. In Cassels E.E.(Ed). *The Heart and Circulation in the Newborn and Infant*. New York: Grune and Stratton.

Capstick, B., Edwards, P. (1991). 'Defensive obstetric practice'. *Lancet* 338, 8770, p.823.

Capsticks Solicitors (1994) 'Capsticks sponsors obstetric research'. *Health Service Journal*. 104, 5398, Special Report - NHS and the Law. Supplement; Capsticks Solicitors, 1-2.

Cario, G. (1985). 'Fetal monitoring'. *Senior Nurse*. Vol. 2, No. 3, pp.14–16.

Carter, B.S., Haverkamp, A.D., Merenstein, G.B. (1993). 'The definition of acute perinatal asphyxia'. *Clinics in Perinatalogy*. 20, 2, pp.287–304.

Castillo, R.A., Devoe, L.D., Arthur, M., Searle, N., Metheny, W., Ruedrich, D.A. (1989) 'The preterm nonstress test: effects of gestational age and length of study'. *American Journal of Obstetrics and Gynaecology*. 160, pp.172 -75.

Chalmers, I., Enkin, M. and Keirse, M.J.N.C. (Eds). (1989). *Effective Care in Pregnancy and Childbirth*. Oxford: Oxford University Press.

Christianson, R.E. (1979). 'Gross differences observed in the placentae of smokers and non-smokers'. *American Journal of Epidemiology* 110, pp. 178–87.

Cohen, W.R. (1988). 'Fetal heart rate monitoring'. in *Current Therapy in Obstetrics*. Charles, D., Glover, D.D. (Eds). Toronto: B.C. Decker Inc.

Cooke, P. (1992). 'Fetal monitoring – a questionable practice?' *Modern Midwife* 12, 2, pp.8–11.

Crowther, C., Enkin, M., Keirse, M.J.N.C., Brown, I. (1989). 'Monitoring the progress in labour'. In: Chalmers, I., Enkin, M., Keirse, M.J.N.C. (Eds). *Effective Care in Pregnancy and Childbirth*. Oxford: Oxford University Press, pp.833–45.

Curzen, P., Bekir, J.S., Patel, M. (1984) 'Reliability of cardiotocography in predicting baby's condition at birth'. *British Medical Journal* 289, 6455, pp.1345–47.

Dawes, G.S. (1993). 'The fetal ECG: accuracy of measurements'. *British Journal of Obstetrics and Gynaecology*. March. Vol. 100 Supplement 9, pp.15-17.

Dawes, G.S., Lobb, M., Moulden, M., Redman, C.W.G., Wheeler, T. (1992). 'Antenatal cardiotocogram quality and interpretation using computers'. *British Journal of Obstetrics and Gynaecology*. 99, pp.791–97.

Dawson, A.J., Middlemiss, C., Coles, E.C., Gough, N.A.J., Jones, M.E. (1989). 'A randomized study of a domiciliary antenatal care scheme: the effect on hospital admissions'. *British Journal of Obstetrics and Gynaecology*, November, Vol. 96, pp.1319–22.

Dennis, J., Johnson, A., Mutch, L., Youdkin, P., Johnson, P. (1989). 'Acid-base status at birth and neurodevelopmental outcome at four and one-half years'. *Americal Journal of Obstetrics and Gynecology* 161, 213–20.

Department of Health (1993). *Changing Childbirth*. Report of the Expert Maternity Group. Chaired by Lady Cumberlege. London: HMSO.

Devoe, L. (1988). 'Antepartum fetal testing'. In: Charles, D., Glover, D. (Eds) *Current Therapy in Obstetrics*. pp.60–67, Toronto: B.C. Decker Inc.

Dijxhoorn, M.J., Visser, G.H.A., Fidler, V.J., Touwen, B.C.L., Huisjes, H.J. (1986) 'Apgar score, meconium and acidaemia at birth in relation to neonatal neurological morbidity in term infants'. *British Journal of Obstetrics and Gynaecology*. 82, pp. 335–59.

Dimond, B. (1990). *Legal Aspects of Nursing*. Hemel Hempstead: Prentice Hall, p.29.

Druzin, M.L., Ikenoue, T., Murata, Y. et al (1979) *A Possible Mechanism for the Increase in FHR Variability Following Hypoxemia*. Presented at the 26th Annual Meeting of Society for Gynecological Investigation, San Diego, California, March 23 1979.

Druzin, M.L. (1989). 'Antepartum fetal heart rate monitoring: state of the art'. *Clinics in Perinatology* 16, 3, pp.661–89.

Druzin, M.L. (1992). *Antepartum Fetal Assessment*. Boston, USA: Blackwell Scientific Publications.

Eganhouse, D.J., Burnside, S.M. (1992). 'Nursing assessment and responsibilities in monitoring the preterm pregnancy'. *The Journal of Obstetric, Gynecological and Neonatal Nursing*. Vol 21, No.5, Sept/Oct, pp.355-62.

Ellison, P.H., Foster, M., Sheridan-Pereira, M., MacDonald, D. (1991) 'Electronic fetal heart monitoring, auscultation and neonatal outcome'. *American Journal of Obstetrics and Gynaecology*. 164, 5, part 1, May, pp.1281–89.

Ennis, M., Clark, A., Grudzinskas, J.G. (1991). 'Change in obstetric practice in response to fear of litigation in the British Isles'. *Lancet* 338, 8767, pp.616–18.

Evans, S. (1992). 'The value of cardiotocograph monitoring in midwifery'. *Midwives Chronicle* 105, 1248, January, pp.4-10.

Evertson, L.R., Gauthier, R.J., Shifrin, B.S., Paul, R.H. (1979). 'Antepartum fetal heart testing'. *Americal Journal of Obstetrics and Gynaecology* 133, pp.29–33.

FIGO (1987). 'Guidelines for the use of fetal monitoring'. *International Journal of Gynaecology and Obstetrics*. 25, pp.1159-67.

Fleischer, A., Schulman, H., Jagani, N., Mitchell, J., Randolph, G. (1982). 'The development of fetal acidosis in the presence of an abnormal fetal heart rate tracing. 1. The average for gestational age fetus'. *American Journal of Obstetrics and Gynecology* 144, pp.55–60.

Flynn, A.M., Kelly, J., Mansfield, H., Needham, P., O'Connor, M., Viego, O. (1982). 'A randomized controlled trial of nonstress antepartum cardiotocography'. *British Journal of Obstetrics and Gynaecology*. 89, pp.427–33.

Freeman, R. (1990). 'Intrapartum fetal monitoring – a disappointing story'. *New England Journal of Medicine* 322, 9, pp.624–26.

Freeman, R.K., Garite, T.J., Nageotte, M.P. (1991). *Fetal Heart Rate Monitoring*. Second edition. Baltimore: Williams and Wilkins.

Garcia, J., Corry, C., MacDonald, D., Elbourne, D., Grant, A. (1985). 'Mothers views of continuous electronic fetal heart monitoring and intermittent auscultation in a randomised controlled trial.' *Birth* 12, pp.79–85.

Gibb, D., Arulkumaran, S. (1992). *Fetal Monitoring in Practice*. Oxford: Butterworth-Heinemann.

Gibb, D.M.F. (1993). 'Measurement of uterine activity in labour - clinical aspects'. *British Journal of Obstetric Gynaecology*. 100 (S9) pp.28-91.

Gibbons, J.M., Nagle, P. (1980). 'Correlation of nonstressed fetal heart rate with sequential contraction stress test'. *Obstetrics and Gynaecology* 55, pp.612–76.

Goodlin, R.C., Lowe, E.W. (1974). 'A functional umbilical cord occlusion heart rate pattern. The significance of overshoot.' *Obstetrics and Gynaecology*. 42, p.27.

Grant, A. (1989). 'Monitoring the fetus during labour'. In: Chalmers, I., Enkin, M., Keirse, M.J.N.C. (Eds). *Effective Care in Pregnancy and Childbirth*. Oxford: Oxford University Press, pp. 846–82.

Grant, A., Mohide, P. (1982). 'Screening and diagnostic test in antenatal care'. In: Enkin, M., Chalmers, I. (Eds). *Effectiveness and Satisfaction in Antenatal Care.* London: William Heinemann.

Grant, A., O'Brien, N., Joy, M.T., Hennesy, E., MacDonald, D. (1989). 'Cerebral palsy among children born during the Dublin randomized trial of intrapartum monitoring', *Lancet* 2, 8674, pp.1233–35.

Hammacher, K., (1969). 'The clinical significance of cardiotocography'. In Huntington P.M., Huter K.A., Saline A. (Eds) *Perinatal Medicine.* Stuttgart: George Thieme Verlagg.

Hammacher, K. (1969). 'The clinical significance of cardiotocography'. In: Huntingford, P.S., Huter, E.A., Saline, E. (Eds). *Perinatal Medicine.* New York: New York Academic Press.

Harvey, C.J. (1989). 'Interpreting the electronic fetal monitor – Strategies for management'. *Journal of Nurse Midwifery* 34, 2, March/April, pp.75–84.

Hon, E.H. (1968). *Atlas of Fetal Heart Rate Patterns.* New Haven: Harty Press.

Hon, E.H., Murata, Y., Zanini, B. et al (1974). 'Continuous microfilm display of the electromechanical intervals of the cardiac cycle'. *Obstetrics and Gynecology,* 43, pp.722–28.

Hull, J., Dodd, K. (1991). 'What is birth asphyxia?' *British Journal of Obstetrics and Gynaecology,* 98, 10, Oct., pp. 953–55.

Itskovitz, J., Goetzman, B.W., Rudolph, A.M. (1982). 'Mechanism of late decelerations of FHR'. *American Journal of Obstetrics and Gynecology,* 142, pp. 66–73.

James, L.S., Yeh, M.N., Morishima, H.O., Daniel, S.S., Caritis, S.N., Niemann, W.H., Indyk, L. (1976). 'Umbilical vein occlusion and transient acceleration of the fetal heart rate. Experimental observations in sub-human primates'. *American Journal of Obstetrics and Gynaecology.* 126, pp.276-83

Johnson, N., Johnson, V.A., Fisher, J., Jobbings, B., Bannister, J., Lilford, R.J. (1991). 'Fetal monitoring with pulse oximetry'. *British Journal of Obstetrics and Gynaecology,* 98, pp.36–41.

Kahn, K.A., Simonson, E. (1957). 'Changes in mean spatial QRS and T vectors and of conventional electrocardiographic items in hard anaerobic work.' *Circulatory Research* 32, pp.725–32.

Keirse, M.J.N.C. (1989). 'Preterm birth'. In: Chalmers, I., Enkin, M., Keirse, M.J.N.C. (Eds). *Effective Care in Pregnancy and Childbirth.* Oxford: Oxford University Press, pp.1270–92.

Kenyon, S. (1994). 'Effects of assessment units on the hospitalization of pregnant women'. *British Journal of Midwifery* . Vol. 2, No. 1, pp.26–28.

Krebs, H.B., Petres, R.E., Dunn, L.J. (1983) 'Fetal heart-rate patterns in the second stage of labor'. *American Journal of Obstetrics and Gynecology.* 140, pp.415-39.

Kubli, F., Kaeser, O., Hinselmann, M. (1969). 'Diagnostic management of chronic placental insufficiency'. In: Pecile, A., Finci, C. (Eds). *The Fetoplacental Unit.* Amsterdam: Exerpta Medica.

Kubli, F.W., Hon, E.H., Khazin, Q.F., Takemura, H. (1969). 'Observations on heart rate and pH in the human fetus at term'. *American Journal of Obstetrics and Gynecology* 104, pp. 1190–206.

Lee, C. et al (1975). 'A study of fetal heart rate acceleration pattern'. *Journal of Obstetrics and Gynaecology,* 45, pp.142–46.

Lotgering, F.K, Wallenburg, H.C.S., Shoulten, H.J.A. (1982). 'Interobserver and intraobserver variation in the assessment of antepartum cardiotocograms'. *AM J Obstet Gynecol* 144, pp.701–50.

MacDonald, D., Grant, A., Sheridan-Pereira, B., Chalmers, I. (1985). 'The Dublin randomised controlled trial of intrapartum fetal heart rate monitoring'. *American Journal of Obstetrics and Gynecology* 152, 5, pp.539–43.

Martin, C.B. (1982). 'Physiology and clinical use of fetal heart rate variability'. *Clinics in Perinatology* 9, 2, pp. 339–52.

Maxwell, D.J., Crawford, D.C., Curry, P.V.M., Tynan, M.J., Allen, L.D. (1988). 'Obstetric importance, diagnosis and management of fetal tachycardias'. *British Medical Journal* 297, pp.107–10.

McNamara, K.W., Russell, V., Johnson, P. (1992). 'Clinical assessment of fetal electrocardiogram monitoring in labour'. *British Journal of Obstetrics and Gynaecology*, 99, pp.32–37.

McNiven, P., Roch, B., Wall, J. (1994). 'Meconium-stained amniotic fluid'. *Modern Midwife.* July, pp.17–20.

Milner, I. (1986). 'Choosing a natural or an active birth'. *Nursing* 3:2, pp.39-45.

Modanlou, H.D., Freeman, R.K. (1982) 'Sinusoidal fetal heart rate pattern: its definition and clinical significance'. *American Journal of Obstetrics and Gynaecology*. 142 pp.1033-38.

Modanlou, H.D., Freeman, R.K., Braly, P. (1977). 'A simple method of fetal and neonatal heart rate beat-to-beat variability quantation: preliminary report'. *American Journal of Obstetrics and Gynecology*. 127, p.861.

Mohide, P., Keirse, M. (1991). 'Method of biophysical assessment'. In: Chalmers, I., Enkin, M., Keirse, M. (Eds). *Effective Care in Pregnancy and Childbirth*. Vol. 1, Parts I–V, Oxford: Oxford University Press.

Murphy, K.W., Chung, D.C., Lilford, R.J., Johnson, N. (1992). 'Do fetal pulse oximetry readings at delivery correlate with cord-blood oxygenation and acidaemia?' *British Journal of Obstetrics and Gynaecology*, 99, pp.735–38.

Murphy, K.W., Johnson, P., Moorcraft, J., Pattinson, R., Russell, V., Turnbull, A. (1990). 'Birth asphyxia and the intrapartum cardiotocograph'. *British Journal of Obstetrics and Gynaecology,* 97, 6, June, pp. 470–79.

Murray, H.G. (1986). 'The fetal electrocardiogram: current clinical development in Nottingham'. *Journal of Perinatal Medicine,* 14, pp.399–404.

Naattgeboren, C. (1989). 'The biology of childbirth'. In: Chalmers, I., Enkin, M., Keirse, M.J.N.C. (Eds). *Effective Care in Pregnancy and Childbirth*. Oxford: Oxford University Press, pp.795–803.

Nielson, P.V., Stigsby, B., Nickelson, C., Nim, J. (1987). 'Intra and inter-observer variability in the assessment of intrapartum cardiotocograms'. *Acta Obstet Gynecol Scand* 66, pp.421–24.

O'Brien, P.M.S., Doyle, P.M., Rolfe, P. (1993). 'Near infrared spectroscopy in fetal monitoring'. *British Journal of Hospital Medicine,* 49, 7, pp.483–87.

Odent, M. (1984). *Birth Reborn*. London: Souvenir Press.

Odent, M. (1994). 'Is electronic fetal monitoring compatible with the art of midwifery?' *Midwifery Matters* Spring Issue 60, p.9.

Olah. K., Henderson, C., Birkbeck, J. (1993). 'Assessment of uterine contractions: midwife or monitor'. *British Journal of Midwifery.* July/August, Vol.1, No.3, pp.111-14, 116-18.

Organ, L.W., Bernstein, A., Smith, K.C., Rowe, I.H. (1974). 'The pre-ejection period of the fetal heart: patterns of change during labor'. *American Journal of Obstetrics and Gynecology*. 120, pp.49–55.

Paine, L.L., Benedict, M.I., Strobino, D.M., Geger, C.L., Larson, E.L. (1992). 'A comparison of the auscultated acceleration test and the nonstress test as predictors of perinatal outcome'. *Nursing Research* 1, 2 Mar-Apr, pp.87–91.

Parer, J.T. (1983). *Handbook of Fetal Heart Rate Monitoring*. Philadelphia: W.B. Saunders.

Paul, R.H., Miller, F.C. (1978). 'Antepartum fetal heart rate monitoring'. *Clinical Obstetrics and Gynaecology* 21, pp.375–84.

Phelan, J. P., Smith, C.V., Broussard, P., Small, M. (1987). 'Amniotic fluid volume assessment using the four quadrant technique in the pregnancy between 36 and 42 weeks gestation'. *Journal Reproductive Medicine* 32, 5, p.40

Pillai, M., Jones, D. (1990). 'The development of fetal heart rate patterns during normal pregnancy'. *Obstetrics and Gynaecology* 76, pp.812–16.

Prentice, A., Lind, T. (1987). 'Fetal heart rate monitoring during labour – too frequent intervention, too little benefit?' *Lancet* ii, 8572, pp.1375–77.

Ramsey, E.M., Corner, G.W., Donner, M.W. (1963). 'Serial and cineradioangiographic visualization of maternal circulation in the primate placenta'. *American Journal of Obstetrics and Gynaecology,* 86, pp. 213–22.

Redman, C.W.G. (1993). 'Communicating the significance of the fetal heart rate record to the user'. *British Journal Obstetrics and Gynaecology*. Vol. 100, Supp. 9, pp.24–27.

Reginald, P.W., Mackinnon, H. (1984). 'Antenatal baseline fetal bradycardia associated with congenital hypothyroidism'. *Journal of Obstetrics and Gynaecology.* 5, pp.40–41.

Richardson, B.S. (1989). 'Fetal adaptive responses to asphyxia'. *Clinics in Perinatology* 16, 20, pp. 595–611.

Robinson, P.L., O'Mullane, N.M., Alderman, B. (1979). 'Prenatal treatment of fetal thyrotoxicosis'. *British Medical Journal* 1, pp.383–84.

Ron M., Adoni A., Hochner-Celnikier D. et al (1980). 'The significance of baseline tachycardia in the post-term fetus'. *International Journal of Gynaecology and Obstetrics.* 18, p.76.

Rosen, K.G., Greene, K.R., Hokegard, K.H., Karlsson, K., Lilja, H., Lindecrantz, K., Kjellmer, I. (1986). 'ST waveform analysis of the fetal ECG – a potent method for fetal surveillance? A presentation of experimental and clinical data'. In: *Cardiovascular and Respiratory Physiology in the Fetus and Neonate.* INSERM/John Libbey Eurotext Ltd 133, pp.67–82.

Rosen, M.G., Dickinson, J.C. (1993). 'The paradox of electronic fetal monitoring: More data may not enable us to predict or prevent infant neurologic morbidity'. *American Journal of Obstetrics and Gynaecology*, 168, 3, pp.745–51.

Rudolph, A. M., Heymann, M.A. (1976). 'Cardiac output in the fetal lamb: the effects of spontaneous and induced changes of heart rate on right and left ventricular output'. *American Journal of Obstetrics and Gynaecology* 124, pp. 183–92.

Ruth, V.J., Ravivio, K.O. (1988). 'Perinatal brain damage: predictive value of metabolic acidosis and Apgar score'. *British Medical Journal* 297, pp.24–27.

Saling E., Schneider, D. (1967). 'Biochemical supervision of the foetus during labour'. *Journal of Obstetrics and Gynaecology of the British Commonwealth.* 74, p.799.

Schifrin, B.S., Clement, D. (1990). 'Why fetal monitoring remains a good idea'. *Contemporary Obstetrics and Gynaecology.* 35, pp.70-86.

Shenker, L. (1973). 'Clinical experience with fetal heart rate monitoring of 1000 patients in labor'. *American Journal of Obstetrics and Gynaecology.* 115, p.1111.

Shy, K.K., Larson, E.B., Luthy, D.A. (1987). 'Evaluating a new technology: The effectiveness of electronic fetal heart rate monitoring'. *Annual Review of Public Health* 8, p.165.

Smith, J.H., Anand, K.J.S., Cotes, P.M. et al (1988). 'Antenatal fetal heart rate variation in relation to the respiratory and metabolic state of the compromised human fetus'. *British Journal of Obstetrics and Gynaecology* 95, pp.980–89.

Smith, J.H., Anand, K.J.S., Cotes, P.M., Dawes, G.S., Harkness, R.A., Howlett, T.A., Rees, L.H., Redman, C.W.G. (1988). 'Antenatal fetal heart rate variation in relation to the respiratory and metabolic status of the compromised human fetus'. *British Journal of Obstetrics and Gynaecology* 95, 980–89.

Spencer, J.A.D., (1989). 'Fetal heart rate variability'. In Studd J. (Ed) *Progress in Obstetrics and Gynaecology.* Chap 7, pp.103-122, Edinburgh: Churchill Livingstone.

Spencer, J.A.D. (Ed). (1992). *Fetal Monitoring.* Oxford: Oxford University Press.

Spencer, J.A.D. (1993). 'Clinical overview of cardiotocography'. *British Journal of Obstetrics and Gynaecology* 100, Suppl. 9, pp.4–7.

Spencer, J.A.D., Johnson, P. (1986). 'FHR variability changes and fetal behavioural cycles in labour'. *British Journal of Obstetrics and Gynaecology* 93, pp.314–21.

Starkman, M. (1976). 'Psychological responses to the use of the fetal monitor during labour.' *Psychosomatic Medicine* 38, 269–77.

Steer, P.J. (1989). 'Intrapartum monitoring in IUGR'. In: Howie, P., Fraser, R. (Eds). *Royal College of Obstetricians and Gynaecologists Study Group on Intrauterine Growth Retardation.* London: Royal College of Obstetricians and Gynaecologists.

Steer, P.J. (1990). 'What determines fetal heart rate?' In: Chamberlain, G. (Ed). *Modern Antenatal Care of the Fetus.* Oxford: Blackwell Scientific Publications, pp.151–61.

Symonds, E.M. (1971). 'Configuration on the fetal electrocardiogram in relation to fetal acid-base balance and plasma electrolytes'. *Journal of Obstetrics and Gynaecology of the British Commonwealth*, 78, pp.957–63.

Symonds, E.M. (1993). 'Litigation and the cardiotocogram'. *British Journal of Obstetrics and Gynaecology* 100, Suppl. 9, March, pp.8–9.

Thacker, S.B. (1992). 'Effectiveness and safety of intrapartum fetal monitoring'. In: Spencer, J.A.D. (Ed). *Fetal Monitoring*. Oxford: Oxford University Press.

Tsechovski, M.S. for the WHO (1993). 'Routine ultrasound scanning during pregnancy'. Letter circulated to all maternity units, ref. HSHCOSPD.DOC. Copenhagen: Regional Office for Europe.

Tucker, S.M. (1992). *Fetal Monitoring*. 2nd edn. Missouri, USA: Mosby-Year Book Inc.

UKCC (1989). *Exercising Accountability*. London: UKCC.

UKCC (1992a). *Code of Professional Conduct*. London: UKCC.

UKCC (1992b). *The Scope of Prefessional Practice*. London: HMSO.

UKCC (1993a). *Standards for Records and Record Keeping*. London: UKCC.

UKCC (1993b). *Midwives Rules*. London: UKCC.

UKCC (1994). *Midwives Code of Practice*. London: UKCC.

Uzan, S., Fouillot, J.P., Sureau, C. (1991). 'Computer analysis of FHR patterns in labour'. In: Spencer, J.A.D. (Ed). *Fetal Monitoring*. Oxford: Oxford University Press.

Van den Berg, P., Schmidt, S., Gesche, J., Saling, E. (1987). 'Fetal distress and the condition of the newborn using cardiotocography and fetal blood analysis during labour'. *British Journal of Obstetrics and Gynaecology*. 94, 1, Jan, pp.72–75.

Wagner, M.G. (1986). 'Birth and Power'. In: Phaff, J.M.L. (Ed). *Perinatal Health Services in Europe: searching for better childbirth*. Beckenham: Croom Helm, for the WHO Regional Office for Europe.

Walker, A.M. (1984). 'Physiological control of the fetal cardiovascular system'. In *Fetal Physiology and Medicine*. Beard R.W. Nathanielsz P.W. (Eds). London: Butterworths. pp.287-316.

Warner, H., Cox, A. (1962). 'A mathematical model to heart rate control by sympathetic and vagus efferent information'. *Journal of Applied Physiology* 17, p.349.

Wheble, A.M., Giller, M.D.G., Spencer, J.A.D., Sykes, G.S. (1989). 'Changes in fetal monitoring in the UK'. *British Journal of Obstetrics and Gynaecology*, 96, 10, Oct. pp.114–47.

Whittle, M.J. (1988). 'Fetal physiology in labour'. In: Chamberlain, G. (Ed). *Contemporary Obstetrics and Gynaecology*. London: Butterworth.

Wigglesworth, J.S., Singer, D.B. (1991). *Textbook Of Fetal And Perinatal Pathology* Vols 1 and 2. Oxford: Blackwell Scientific Publications.

Williams, C.E., Mallard, C., Tan, W., Gluckman, P.D. (1993). 'Pathophysiology of perinatal asphyxia'. *Clinics in Perinatology* 20, 2, June, pp.305–25.

Wood, P.L., Dobbie, H.G. (1989). *Electronic Fetal Heart Rate Monitoring*. Basingstoke: MacMillan Press.

World Health Organisation Regional Office for Europe (1985). *Having a Baby in Europe*. Copenhagen: WHO.

Young, B.K., Katz, M.,Wilson, S.J. (1980). 'Sinusoidal fetal heart rate'. In. Clinical significance. *American Journal of Obstetrics and Gynecology*. 136, pp.587-593.

Recommended Further Reading

Anthony, M.Y., Levene, M.I. (1990). 'An assessment of the benefits of intrapartum fetal monitoring.' *Developmental Medicine and Child Neurology* 32, 6, pp.547–53.

Balen, A.H. (1993). 'The value of cardiotocography for intrapartum monitoring.' *British Journal of Midwifery* 1, 4, Sept., pp.174–76.

Chalmers, I., Enkin, M., Keirse, M.J.N.C. (1989). *Effective Care in Pregnancy and Childbirth*. Oxford: Oxford University Press.

Cooke, P. (1992). 'Fetal monitoring – A Questionable Practice?' *Modern Midwife* 12, 2, April, pp.8–11.

Curzen, P., Bekir, J.S., Patel, M. (1984). 'Reliability of cardiotocography in predicting a baby's condition at birth.' *British Medical Journal* 289, 6455, pp.1345–47.

Druzin, M.L. (1992). *Antepartum Fetal Assessment*. Oxford: Blackwell Scientific Publications.

Eganhouse, D.J., Burnside, S.M. (1992). 'Nursing assessment and responsibilities in monitoring the preterm pregnancy'. *Journal of Obstetrics Gynaecology and Neonatal Nursing* 21, 5, Sept/Oct, pp.355-63.

Ellison, P.H., Foster, M., Sheridan-Pereira, M., MacDonald, D. (1991). 'Electronic fetal heart monitoring, auscultation, and neonatal outcome.' *American Journal of Obstetrics and Gynecology* 164, 5, Part 1, pp.1281-89.

Evans, S. (1992). 'The value of cardiotocograph monitoring in midwifery'. *Midwives Chronicle* 105, 1248, pp.4-10.

Fox, R. (1989). 'Cerebral palsy, intrapartum care and a shot in the foot'. *Lancet* ii, 8674, pp. 1251–52 (editorial).

Freeman, R. (1990). 'Intrapartum fetal monitoring - a disappointing story.' *New England Journal of Medicine* 322, 9, March, pp.624-26.

Freeman, R.K., Garite, T.J., Nageotte, M.P. (1991). *Fetal Heart Rate Monitoring*. Baltimore: Williams and Wilkins.

Gauge, S.M., Henderson, C. (1992). *CTG Made Easy*. Edinburgh: Churchill Livingstone.

Gibb, D., Arulkumaran, S. (1992). 'Control of the fetal heart'. In: *Fetal Monitoring in Practice*. Chapter 4. Oxford: Butterworth Heinemann.

Grant, A., O'Brien, J., Joy, M.T., Hennesy, E., MacDonald, D. (1989). 'Cerebral palsy among children born during the Dublin randomised trial of intrapartum monitoring'. *Lancet* ii, pp.1233-35.

Hillan, E. (1991). 'Electronic fetal monitoring - more problems than benefits?' *MIDIRS Midwifery Digest* 1, 3, pp.249-51.

Hull, J., Dodd, K. (1991). 'What is birth asphyxia?' *British Journal of Obstetrics and Gynaecology* 98, 10, Oct, pp.953-55.

MacDonald, D., Grant, A., Sheridan-Pereira, B., Chalmers, I. (1985). 'The Dublin randomised controlled trial of intrapartum fetal heart rate monitoring'. *American Journal of Obstetrics and Gynecology* 152, 5, pp.539-43.

Murphy, K.W., Johnson, P., Moorcraft, J., Pattinson, R., Russell, V., Turnbull, A. (1990). 'Birth asphyxia and the intrapartum cardiotocograph'. *British Journal of Obstetrics and Gynaecology* 97, 6, June, pp.470-79.

Murphy-Black, T. (1991). 'Fetal monitoring in labour'. *Nursing Times* 87, 28, pp.58-59.

Richardson, B.S. (1989). 'Fetal adaptive responses to asphyxia'. *Clinics in Perinatology* 16, 20, pp.595-611.

Rosen, M.G., Dickinson, J.C. (1993). 'The paradox of electronic fetal monitoring: more data may not enable us to predict or prevent infant neurologic morbidity'. *American Journal of Obstetrics and Gynecology* 168, 3, pp.745-51.

Schifrin, B.S. (1990). *Exercises in Fetal Monitoring*. St Louis, Missouri: Mosby Year Book.

Schifrin, B.S. (1990). *Exercises in Fetal Monitoring*. London: Wolfe Publishing.

Sheil, O. (1993). 'Asphyxia, acidaemia, Apgars and the fetal heart'. *Contemporary Reviews in Obstetrics and Gynaecology* 5, Oct., pp.202-206.

Spencer, J.A.D. (1993). 'Clinical overview of cardiotocography'. *British Journal of Obstetrics and Gynaecology* 100, Suppl. 9, March, pp.4-7.

Steer, P.J. (1990). 'What determines fetal heart rate?' In: Chamberlain, G. (Ed). *Modern Antenatal Care of the Fetus*. Oxford: Blackwell Scientific Publications, pp.151-61.

Symonds, E.M. (1993). 'Litigation and the cardiotocogram'. *British Journal of Obstetrics and Gynaecology* 100, Suppl. 9, March, pp.8-9.

Whittle, M.J. (1988). 'Fetal physiology in labour'. In: Chamberlain, G. (Ed). *Contemporary Obstetrics and Gynaecology*. London: Butterworth.

Wood, P.L., Dobbie, H.G. (1989). *Electronic Fetal Heart Rate Monitoring: A Practical Guide*. Basingstoke: Macmillan.

Index